KIDNEY
AND URINARY TRACT
INFECTIONS

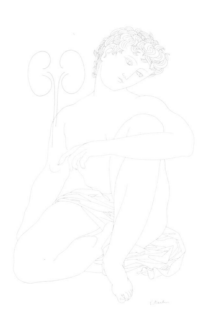

Published by the LILLY RESEARCH LABORATORIES
Indianapolis, Indiana

CONTRIBUTORS
E. Lovell Becker, M.D., F.A.C.P.
Professor of Medicine
Cornell University Medical College
New York, New York

Lawrence R. Freedman, M.D.
Professor of Medicine
Yale University School of Medicine
New Haven, Connecticut

Robert M. Kark, M.D., F.R.C.P.
Professor of Medicine
Rush Medical College
Chicago, Illinois

Richard H. Kessler, M.D.
Professor of Medicine
Northwestern University Medical School
Chicago, Illinois

CONSULTING EDITOR
E. Lovell Becker, M.D.

EDITORS
Mitchell Kory, Ph.D.
S. O. Waife, M.D., F.A.C.P.

SENIOR ART DIRECTOR
C. E. Hammond

KIDNEY AND URINARY TRACT INFECTIONS

Contents

Kidney and Urinary Tract Infections

1
Introduction

For a long time the kidneys have been the subject of varying opinions, some even having regarded them as superfluous and unnecessary, a thought which is certainly not a tribute to nature. More recently, however, because of their wonderful structure, and because of the very necessary function attributed to them, they have attained a place among the important parts of the body.

—*Marcello Malpighi (1628–1694)*

A few years ago there would have been little interest in a monograph on kidney and urinary tract infections. The clinical picture of acute pyelonephritis seemed clear, and its progression to chronic pyelonephritis was easily identified by pathologists and generally accepted without challenge.[1]

Today, we know that the entity called *acute pyelonephritis* may be only the "top of the iceberg" of urinary tract infections; that morphologic criteria for the diagnosis of chronic pyelonephritis are both controversial and nonspecific; and that documentation establishing that advanced renal disease is caused by repeated urinary infections has proved to be a most difficult task.[2-4] In the opinion of many clinicians, the ensuing complexity and confusion have been responsible for overtreatment of inconsequential illnesses and lack of sufficient concern for potentially serious infections (Figure 1).

Helkiah: Microcosmographia: A Description of the Body of Man. London, 1615. (Courtesy of the Lilly Library, Indiana University, Bloomington, Indiana)

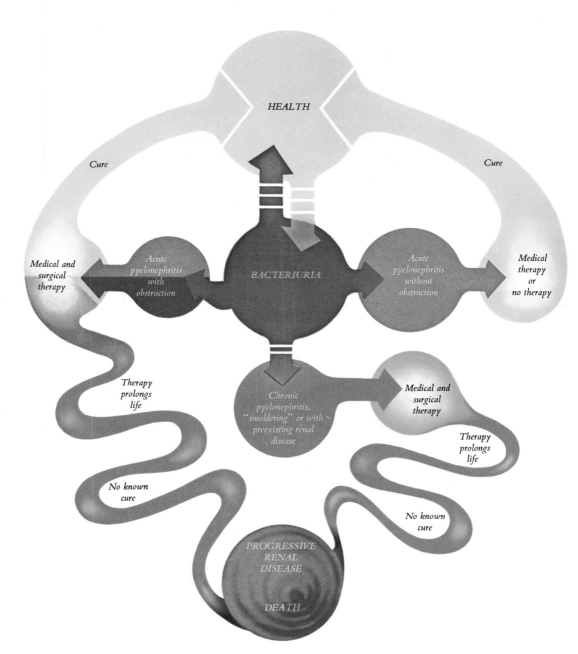

Figure 1. Interrelationships of urinary tract infections. The central position of bacteriuria in the chart emphasizes its generally accepted role in the development of acute pyelonephritis, either with or without obstruction. Return to health from acute pyelonephritis with therapy (or even in its absence) is the usual occurrence. When obstruction is present, however, appropriate therapy may lead to health, but it does not do so in a substantial number of cases. Instead, life is prolonged, but renal disease continues. The relationship of bacteriuria to chronic pyelonephritis is not clear, as the striped arrow indicates. In contrast, there is no suggestion that acute pyelonephritis precedes chronic pyelonephritis. Therapy in chronic pyelonephritis may prolong life but does not prevent death due to renal failure.

The pathway from health to bacteriuria and back may be traveled repeatedly, and the striped arrows indicate this without implying that all the factors are understood or even known.

DEFINITIONS

Terminology in this field is frequently ambiguous and is not standardized. Accordingly, the terms used in this book are defined in the following way.

Bacteriuria means bacteria in the urine. Since bacteria are not filtered from the bloodstream by the kidney, urine from the renal pelves, ureters, and bladder should be sterile when conditions are normal. Thus, bacteria in any number detected in urine from these sources is indicative of some abnormality. The anterior urethra, on the other hand, normally contains bacteria on its mucosal surface, and a voided urine sample will always contain bacteria.[5] Therefore, development of the methodology which made it possible to draw inferences about the bacterial content of *bladder* urine by study of cultures of *voided* urine was a major advance. The wide application of these methods is responsible for the vast amount of information which is accumulating at a rapid rate.[6,7] Bacteriuria may or may not be accompanied by other abnormal urinary constituents; it may or may not occur in association with symptoms of illness, and it may or may not be detected in persons with renal disease.

Bacteriuria is indicative of one of the most common infections seen by a wide variety of physicians. Because the symptoms produced by these infections vary so greatly, it is important to examine carefully any evidence that the association of illness with bacteriuria is causal. For example, patients with asymptomatic bacteriuria may develop pain in the right lower quadrant and be found to have appendicitis; some patients with bacteriuria and pain in the right upper quadrant will be found to have gall-bladder disease. Similarly, patients with renal disease of any kind (nephrosclerosis, glomerulonephritis) may have bacteriuria which has played no role or an apparently insignificant one in the pathogenesis of the renal damage.

Urinary tract infection is the term reserved by some authors for bacteriuria associated with either symptoms or signs of infection within the urinary tract. It is, however, most difficult to define the symptoms or to state the precise number of white cells or red cells or the amount of protein which must be found in the urine in order to establish infection. In addition, the requirement that signs or symptoms of infection be present suggests that subjects with bacteriuria alone do not have an infection, a thesis difficult to substantiate. For these reasons, in this book *bacteriuria* and *urinary tract infection* are considered synonymous but are employed with the full realization that tissue infection may exist at any level of the urinary tract and yet not be apparent.

The terms "cystitis" and "pyelitis" should be replaced by the designation "urinary tract infection" with an indication of the portion of the urinary tract responsible for symptoms. Accordingly, "cystitis" is a urinary tract infection with lower-urinary-tract symptoms. Such a description, in contrast to former terminology, does not imply that the infection is confined to a zone of the urinary system which happens to be symptomatic.

Acute pyelonephritis is used to designate findings of acute infection in the renal *parenchyma*. Clinically, the term is used for patients believed to have kidney infection with signs and symptoms of acute illness. The typical picture includes fever, chills, flank pain and tenderness, leukocytosis, bacteriuria, pyuria, and, often, symptoms of lower-urinary-tract inflammation, such as dysuria and frequency of urination.

Pyelonephritis is taken to mean renal parenchymal disease caused by bacterial infection in the kidney and present now or at some time in the past. Urinary tract infection may or may not be detected concurrently. The severity, type, and number of symptoms and signs of renal disease occur according to the amount of renal function which has been lost.

Chronic pyelonephritis has precisely the same meaning. It is essential to distinguish chronic urinary tract infection from chronic pyelonephritis. The former refers only to the prolonged presence of bacteriuria, whereas the latter requires renal disease to be detected and infection to have been important at some time in its pathogenesis.

Chronic interstitial nephritis describes the sites of renal disease without specifying its cause. Thus, when due to bacterial infection, chronic interstitial nephritis is synonymous with chronic pyelonephritis. It is important to emphasize that there are many causes of chronic interstitial nephritis, but all produce changes which are morphologically indistinguishable from those due to infection.[4,8]

A summary of these definitions appears at the end of the chapter in Box 1.

THE PROBLEMS

Surveys of large "normal" populations have uncovered a remarkable prevalence of urinary tract infections among women. Infections are found in about 1 percent of schoolgirls, but the incidence increases with age (depending on the population studied) and reaches a peak of 10 to 12 percent in women over sixty (Figure 2). In contrast, infections are uncommon in men, with a prevalence of about 1 percent at the age of sixty. These data appear in Figure 3.[9-11]

Very little is known about the natural history of these infections. In general, they carry

Figure 2. The frequency of urinary tract infections in rural and urban Jamaican women.[10]

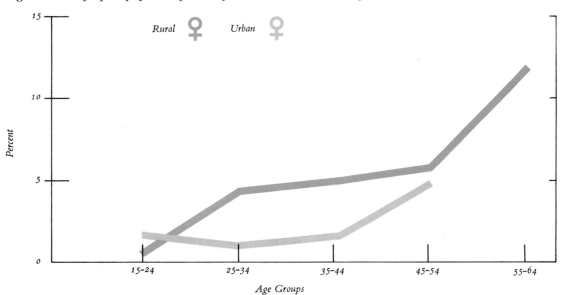

the greatest risk to health when they are accompanied by underlying abnormalities of the urinary tract (cystic change of the kidneys, stone, or obstruction) or when other diseases (diabetes mellitus, nephrosclerosis, and sickle-cell disorders) are present which by themselves are capable of producing kidney or urinary tract damage (Figure 4).

Some data suggest that urinary infections during pregnancy predispose toward premature births.[12] This subject is controversial, however, since the increased risk of prematurity may be related to underlying renal disease of which the urinary infection is only a reflection.

It is not easy to establish the cause of significant renal disease when, on pathological grounds from biopsy material or at autopsy, it is identified as chronic interstitial nephritis. Traditionally, this type of kidney disease was loosely referred to as "chronic pyelonephritis." Investigations of possible causes have revealed very little to support the view that bacterial infection plays an important role in its pathogenesis.[4] Since this is a difficult problem to resolve retrospectively, however, it must be put aside until considerably more information has been collected and analyzed.

Unfortunately, both physician and patient are caught in this speculative maze. If one grants that urinary infections are common, and experience certainly bears this out, how are such infections to be considered? Are they a serious hazard in all patients or only in some, or should they take their place among a long list of chronic diseases which require observation and management but are not immediate threats to survival?

The information available at present favors the latter view provided the infection is not associated with underlying diseases of the urinary tract or diseases which have the capacity to injure the urinary tract (Figure 4).[4]

Although many questions cannot be an-

Figure 3. The frequency of urinary tract infections in Japanese men and women.[11]

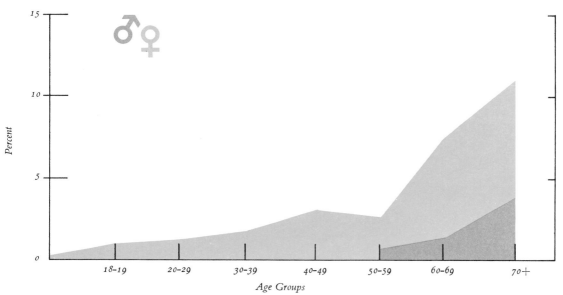

swered until more is learned, some of the controversy can be resolved by examination of available information. The purpose of this monograph is to deal with the issues, to distinguish what is known and what is not, and to distill from the fermentation mixture concepts which physicians will find useful in patient management.

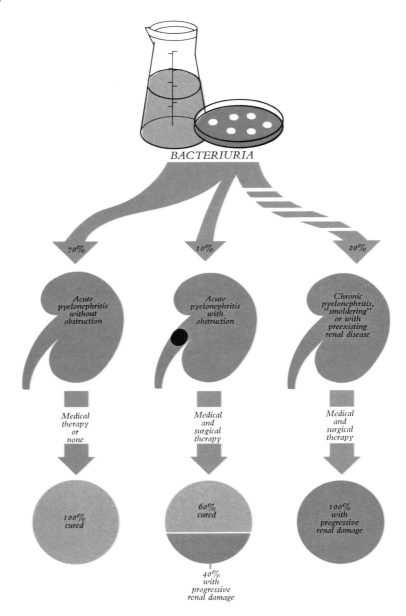

Figure 4. The incidence of bacteriuria (in percent) and the effect of therapy on the clinical course of kidney infections. The striped arrow indicates the uncertain relationship between bacteriuria and chronic pyelonephritis.

BOX 1
SUMMARY OF DEFINITIONS

Bacteriuria— Any bacteria in urine uncontaminated by normal urethral flora.

Urinary Tract Infection— Bacteriuria with or without signs or symptoms of inflammation.

Asymptomatic Bacteriuria— Bacteriuria unaccompanied by clinical symptoms.

Bacteriuria with Urgency, Frequency, and Dysuria— Symptoms suggest infection in lower urinary tract, i.e., "cystitis."

Bacteriuria with Back Pain, Chills, and Fever— Symptoms suggest infection in upper urinary tract, i.e., "acute pyelonephritis" (formerly "pyelitis").

Acute Pyelonephritis— Bacteriuria, with or without lower-urinary-tract symptoms, but with chills, fever, and flank pain and tenderness.

Pyelonephritis, or Chronic Pyelonephritis — Renal disease believed to be caused by bacterial infection in the kidney, either past or present.

Chronic Interstitial Nephritis— Inflammatory changes involving tubules and interstitium most severely; generally sparing of glomeruli. Due to various causes but, when caused by infection, synonymous with pyelonephritis.

BIBLIOGRAPHY

1. Weiss, S., and Parker, F., Jr.: Pyelonephritis: Its Relation to Vascular Lesions and to Arterial Hypertension, Medicine, *18*:221, 1939.

2. Heptinstall, R. H.: The Limitations of the Pathological Diagnosis of Chronic Pyelonephritis, in Renal Disease, Ed. 2 (edited by D. A. K. Black), p. 350. Oxford: Blackwell Scientific Publications, 1967.

3. Beeson, P. B.: Urinary Tract Infection and Pyelonephritis, in Renal Disease, Ed. 2 (edited by D. A. K. Black), p. 382. Oxford: Blackwell Scientific Publications, 1967.

4. Freedman, L. R.: Chronic Pyelonephritis at Autopsy, Ann. Int. Med., *66*:697, 1967.

5. Stamey, T. A., Govan, D. E., and Palmer, J. M.: The Localization and Treatment of Urinary Tract Infections: The Role of Bactericidal Urine Levels as Opposed to Serum Levels, Medicine, *44*:1, 1965.

6. Kass, E. H.: The Role of Asymptomatic Bacteriuria in the Pathogenesis of Pyelonephritis, in Biology of Pyelonephritis (edited by E. L. Quinn and E. H. Kass), p. 399. Boston: Little, Brown & Company, 1960.

7. Turck, M., Ronald, A. R., and Petersdorf, R. G.: Relapse and Reinfection in Chronic Bacteriuria. II. The Correlation between Site of Infection and Pattern of Recurrence in Chronic Bacteriuria, New England J. Med., *278*:422, 1968.

8. Freedman, L. R.: Pyelonephritis and Urinary Tract Infection, in Diseases of the Kidney (edited by M. B. Strauss and L. G. Welt), p. 469. Boston: Little, Brown & Company, 1963.

9. Kunin, C. M., Deutscher, R., and Paquin, A., Jr.: Urinary Tract Infection in School Children: An Epidemiologic, Clinical and Laboratory Study, Medicine, *43*:91, 1964.

10. Miall, W. E., Kass, E. H., Ling, J., and Stuart, K. L.: Factors Influencing Arterial Pressure in the General Population in Jamaica, Brit. M. J., *2*:497, 1962.

11. Freedman, L. R., Phair, J. P., Seki, M., Hamilton, H. B., and Nefzger, M. D.: The Epidemiology of Urinary Tract Infections in Hiroshima, Yale J. Biol. & Med., *37*:262, 1965.

12. Norden, C. W., and Kass, E. H.: Bacteriuria of Pregnancy— A Critical Appraisal, Ann. Rev. Med., *19*: 431, 1968.

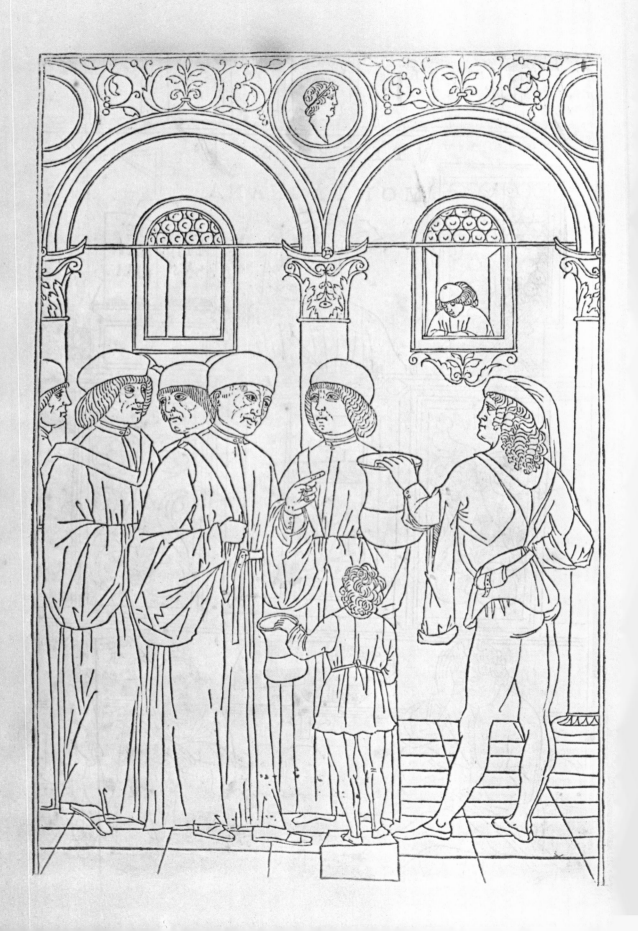

2
The Causes of Urinary Infections

Careful clinical observation and experiments in animals have contributed a great deal of knowledge in the past few years to our understanding of the pathogenesis of urinary tract infection and pyelonephritis.

TYPES OF ORGANISMS

The bacteria commonly responsible for infections in the urinary system are *Escherichia coli*, one or more species of *Klebsiella*, *Enterobacter*, *Proteus*, and *Pseudomonas*, and various enterococci, all normal constituents of the fecal flora.

Figure 5. Causative organisms in acute urinary tract infections in patients without obstruction who have not been treated with antimicrobial agents or subjected to urologic procedures.

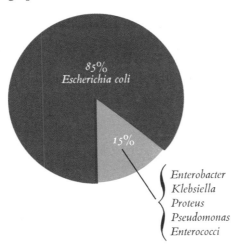

85%
Escherichia coli

15%

}
Enterobacter
Klebsiella
Proteus
Pseudomonas
Enterococci

PATHWAYS BY WHICH BACTERIA ENTER THE URINARY TRACT

The Ascending Route—There is considerable clinical evidence[1] to suggest that the ascent of bacteria within the urethra represents the most common pathway of infection of the urinary tract (Figures 6 and 6a). In the male, the length of the urethra and the antibacterial properties of prostatic secretion are effective barriers to invasion by this route.[4] It has been proposed that these two factors may explain why males have a much lower incidence of urinary tract infections than do females. The common onset of urinary tract infections at the time of marriage and in association with sexual activity clearly implicates the ascending urethral pathway in pathogenesis.

Figure 6. The ascending route of infection. Pathogenic bacteria from external sources ascend the urethra and the ureters to cause bacteriuria.

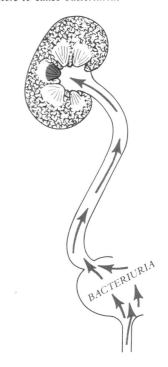

BACTERIURIA

These organisms are not equally significant in the etiology of urinary tract infections. *Esch. coli* is the causative organism in about 85 percent of acute infections of the bladder and kidneys in patients in whom no obstruction exists and neither antimicrobial agents nor instruments have been used (Figure 5). In contrast, patients who have been treated with antimicrobial drugs or who have been subjected to urologic procedures are more likely to have *Proteus, Pseudomonas,* or enterococci as the offending organism.[1-3]

The percent of all urinary tract infections caused by the staphylococcus is small.[1-3] *Staphylococcus aureus* should be detected in large numbers in repeated specimens of urine before it is thought to cause a urinary tract infection. In addition, a primary source of infection (osteomyelitis or abscess) should be searched for elsewhere in the body.

In rare instances, kidney and urinary tract infections are caused by fungi, *Salmonella,* and tubercle bacilli.

Fecal Soiling—Probably the major way in which bacteria are brought to the urinary tract, both in children and in adults, is by fecal soiling of the urethral meatus.

Urethrovesical Reflux—When intrabladder pressure increases suddenly in normal women, as during coughing, urine may be squeezed out of the bladder into the urethra (Figure 7). The urine may then flow back into the bladder when pressures return to normal and, in this way, wash bacteria from the anterior portions of the urethra into the bladder (Figure 7a). This reflux also may be caused by sudden interruption of urination in normal subjects and by hesitant or intermittent voiding due to dysfunction of the bladder neck or urethra.

Figure 6a. Bacteriuria may be maintained by "seeding" of urine from foci of infection in the kidney.

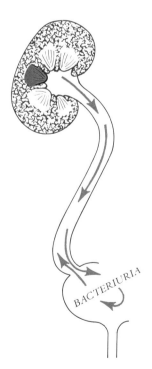

Figure 7. Urethrovesical reflux. Increase of pressure on the bladder forces urine into the urethra. (The dashed line indicates position of bladder before the pressure, represented by arrows, was applied.)

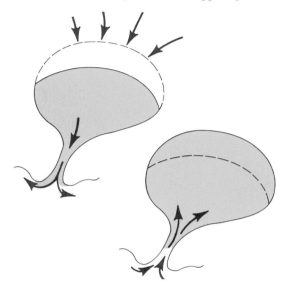

Figure 7a. When pressure returns to normal, urine that has bathed the anterior contaminated portions of the urethra washes bacteria into the bladder.

Instrumentation—The spreading of potentially pathogenic bacteria via instruments is a very important cause of infection because it is common and usually preventable. Typical acute urinary tract infections and pyelonephritis often follow the use of a catheter or cystoscope.[5] For this reason, bladder catheterization solely for the purpose of obtaining a urine specimen is to be condemned. Infections due to *Pseudomonas* are almost all confined to patients who have had instrumentation. This organism is present in feces, but it is also found in tap water and is resistant to many commonly used sterilizing agents. Urinary tract infections contracted in the hospital are usually due to *Enterobacter*, *Proteus*, and the enterococci and appear to be passed from person to person through hands, catheters, bedpans, and instruments. The problem is considered analogous to "hospital staphylococcus" infections.

Blood and Lymph—Infection of the kidney via the bloodstream is unusual but it is to be strongly suspected in cases of staphylococcus urinary infections. In these instances, the kidney infection is likely to be secondary to infection elsewhere in the body. The lymphatic system is frequently mentioned as a possible pathway of infection, but there is little evidence to support this.

Prostate and Paraurethral Glands—Recent studies have emphasized chronic asymptomatic infection of the prostate in men and paraurethral glands in women as possible sources of recurrent urinary infections. These indolent infections are particularly troublesome because antibiotics are characteristically ineffective.[6]

THE FATE OF BACTERIA IN THE BLADDER

Removal of Bacteria—Under normal circumstances, after large bacterial inocula (i.e., 10 to 100 million organisms) reach the bladder urine, they are promptly eliminated. The mechanisms within the bladder lumen responsible for this action are complex and are not adequately understood. Possible factors are (1) ability of urine either to support growth of bacteria or to destroy them, (2) effectiveness of antibacterial properties of the bladder mucosa, (3) efficiency of phagocytosis and availability of substances which enhance or interfere with this process, and (4) removal of bacteria by urination.

All cannot be of equal importance. For instance, voiding is not a very efficient mechanism for ridding the bladder of bacteria; a

film of urine always remains behind, and ample time exists for rapid multiplication before the next voiding. In contrast, the antibacterial properties of the bladder mucosa may be important in maintaining sterility.[7,8]

It is not known how these forces interact, nor is it possible to identify abnormal mechanisms in the majority of patients.

However, the delicacy of the balance between host defenses and bacterial multiplication is illustrated by experiments in animals. The inoculation of 10 to 100 million *Esch. coli* into the bladder lumen is followed by prompt clearance of the organisms and sterilization of the urine. Under circumstances of chronic water diuresis, however, as few as ten bacteria can multiply rapidly and persist for prolonged periods.[9] Thus, susceptibility to urinary infection may be compounded a million times by increased water intake.

It is not known whether similar factors operate in man. Nevertheless, these experiments suggest that even the relatively nontoxic and temporary condition produced by excessive water intake may be sufficient to alter the interaction between bacteria in the bladder lumen and host defense mechanisms. The delicate balance between these opposing forces may be upset by many circumstances to produce important clinical consequences. For example, the risk of producing urinary tract infection in most outpatients by a single catheterization of the bladder is very low—i.e., 1 to 3 percent.[5] In contrast, bedridden hospitalized patients, often aged and usually with other complicating diseases, are probably much more susceptible to infection following catheterization.

Bladder Emptying—According to clinical observation, inability to empty the bladder completely with each voiding is one of the most important factors interfering with clearance of bacteria from the bladder lumen. This does not mean, however, that all patients with residual urine should be subjected to operative attempts at repair. If the patient is already infected, the residual urine may well be a result of the infection (i.e., inability to void completely may be due to edema of the bladder neck or dysuria). If no infection is present, considerable judgment must be exercised in determining whether the risk of introducing infection (especially in a patient with increased susceptibility) outweighs the danger of sterile residual urine. Many patients have persistent infection without residual urine. Thus, elimination of residual urine in cases of persistent infection may not result in cure of the infection in all patients.

Vesicoureteral Reflux—The efficiency of bladder emptying is impaired by vesicoureteral reflux. The mechanism differs from those mentioned previously because there may be no bladder outlet obstruction. When vesicoureteral reflux occurs, urine goes up the ureters during voiding and returns to the bladder when voiding has stopped (Figures

8 and 8a). Therefore, residual urine results from incompetent vesicoureteral valve action due to edema and inflammation caused by infection. Surgical repair should be attempted only when significant reflux (endangering renal function) persists despite four to six months of successful sterilization of the urine. After successful antibiotic therapy, even marked degrees of hydroureter and hydronephrosis may disappear if these changes were caused by reflux secondary to infection.[10]

In recent years, considerable attention has been directed to the problem of vesicoureteral reflux. When demonstrated by currently available radiologic technics, vesicoureteral reflux is definitely an abnormal finding. It must be emphasized, however, that, except when there is gas in the urinary tract, a direct fluid connection between the renal pelvis and the bladder urine is always present. Studies by hydraulic engineers as well as clinical observations support the view that, even under normal conditions, particles may make their way up the ureter against the flow of urine during normal ureteral peristalsis. In one sense, then, vesicoureteral reflux may be

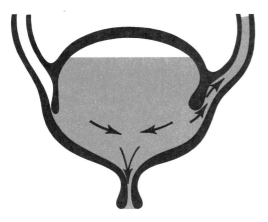

Figure 8. Vesicoureteral reflux. During voiding, urine is forced up the ureter if the vesicoureteral valve is impaired and cannot "shut" tightly.

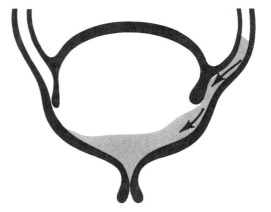

Figure 8a. When voiding ceases, the urine "refluxed" into the ureter returns to the bladder, and thus a pool of residual urine is produced; i.e., voiding never completely empties the bladder.

a normal and continuous occurrence. The abnormality which this term connotes is probably a matter of degree, depending on quantitative judgments. It is well known that successful demonstration of reflux by x-ray depends on many technical factors. Even with standardized technics, it may not be demonstrable in a single patient from one day to the next. All of these facets of the problem must be considered in assessing the chances for success or failure of any proposed therapy.[11]

Aging—One of the least controversial yet inexplicable features of urinary tract infection is the remarkable increase in its prevalence with advancing age. This age distribution has been recognized only recently[12-14] (see page 10). It is particularly interesting because it has upset the traditional view which holds that urinary tract infections occur most often in young women during the period of childbearing. Although data are sparse, the discrepancy between past clinical experience and modern studies cannot be explained by differences in the symptoms, clinical course, or response to therapy of the different age groups.

Blood Pressure—Surveys of large groups of normal women have revealed that persons with positive urine cultures have somewhat higher mean blood pressure than noninfected women in the same population.[12-14] The significance of this small difference in blood pressure is not known, and it is unresolved whether urinary tract infections predispose to higher blood pressure or whether subjects with higher blood pressure are more susceptible to urinary infections. Experiments in animals have dealt with increased susceptibility of the kidney to infection when the blood pressure is raised. In addition, when pyelonephritis is induced experimentally in hypertensive animals, blood pressure increases. As a rule, however, experimentally induced pyelonephritis produces no significant elevation of blood pressure in normal animals until renal insufficiency occurs.

Upper Tract Obstruction—Most upper tract obstructions (i.e., of the ureter and renal pelvis) are sterile, and perhaps all would be if they occurred in patients who did not have bacteria in the bladder urine. There is no evidence that such obstructive lesions make it easier for bacteria to invade the bladder cavity. On the other hand, once bacteria have been introduced into the urinary tract, the presence of an obstructive lesion enormously increases the risk of serious renal destruction by the acute infection. It is of great importance, therefore, to consider carefully the dangers and possible advantages of procedures which may infect sterile urinary obstruction.[15] It is often stated that bladder urine may be sterile despite infection above a ureteral obstructive lesion. If this occurs at all, it must be extraordinarily uncommon.

Diabetes—In diabetes mellitus, the antibacterial defense mechanisms are adversely affected.[16] Furthermore, diabetics are often subjected to urethral catheterization during management of diabetic acidosis and autonomic neuropathy of the bladder. For these reasons, it might be anticipated that urinary infections are more common and more severe in diabetics than in nondiabetics. However, in studies of diabetics carefully matched with controls of the same age, no significant differences appeared in the prevalence of bacteriuria.[17] (For further discussion, see under Glucose and Other Reducing Substances, page 39.) The acute infections associated with papillary necrosis are found in diabetics, but they are relatively uncommon considering the number of diabetics with urinary infections. Furthermore, in studies of diabetic kidneys at autopsy, it has not been possible to distinguish the interstitial nephritis of diabetic nephropathy from similar changes which might be due to infection.[18]

Nevertheless, diabetics have special problems with urinary tract infections. These infections may precipitate acidosis and coma, and they may lead to the development of acute papillary necrosis of the kidney, an unusual but life-threatening variety of acute pyelonephritis.

Pregnancy—It is often stated that bacteriuria is more common during pregnancy. However, numerous surveys of pregnant women show that the incidence of urinary tract infection is within the range known to exist in nonpregnant women of the same age.[3] The data are surprising, since it is generally believed that susceptibility to a variety of infections is increased by pregnancy.

About 40 percent of pregnant women with bacteriuria will develop symptomatic acute pyelonephritis if untreated.[3] It is not known whether the incidence of pyelonephritis would be greater or less in nonpregnant women followed in the same way for the same length of time. The ureteral dilatation which occurs during childbirth provides fertile ground for serious infections, and clinical experience attests to the unusual severity of infections at this time. In addition, there are conflicting data concerning the effect of bacteriuria during pregnancy on birth weight and viability of the fetus.[3] More work is needed to establish the facts, but, in the meantime, apprehension of possible risk to mother and child continues and prompts attempts to control infections during pregnancy. The potential danger of such a course

lies in the administration of drugs which may adversely affect the fetus.

Preexisting Renal Disease—Bacteriuria in the presence of underlying renal disease is a serious problem requiring the thoughtful attention of the physician. It is important to keep the infection from causing further renal damage, yet care must be used in the administration of antimicrobial drugs which may be nephrotoxic.

The effect of preexisting renal disease on the development of bacteriuria is unknown. The problem is complex. Data are needed on prevalence of bacteriuria in patients with renal disease as compared with appropriate controls—i.e., subjects of the same age and sex without renal disease. Furthermore, to make the comparison valid, an assessment of instrumentation is also required, because patients with renal disease are subjected to instrumentation, both for diagnostic and therapeutic purposes, with greater frequency than are those without renal disease.

FACTORS IN THE MULTIPLICATION OF BACTERIA

Extrarenal Urinary Obstruction—Our knowledge of the factors which influence bacterial multiplication in the kidney comes mostly from recent animal experiments.[1] The effect of urinary obstruction, however, was recognized clinically in the late nineteenth century and confirmed promptly in animal studies.[19]

In the absence of extrarenal obstruction, pyelonephritis remains confined to a wedge-shaped zone of kidney with the apex in the medulla (Figure 9). However, in the presence of complete extrarenal obstruction, as by stone or tumor, the acute infection spreads throughout the entire kidney. The destruc-

Figure 9. In the absence of obstruction, there is usually no lateral spread of the infection.

Figure 9a. With obstruction, the infection spreads throughout the entire parenchyma.

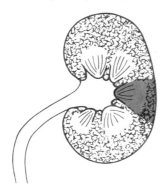

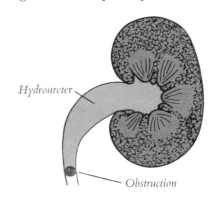

Hydroureter

Obstruction

tion of the kidney under these circumstances may be rapid and complete (Figure 9a).[20]

There is no argument about the therapy in complete urinary obstruction. An attempt must be made to repair the obstruction or total loss of the kidney will result.

When the urinary obstruction is partial, the therapy which should be attempted is less certain. The need for repair must be clearly demonstrated before the patient is subjected to a procedure which may not succeed—or succeed only partially—and which may contaminate tissues already very susceptible to bacterial invasion.

Partial obstruction of the urinary tract in animals increases their susceptibility to pyelonephritis to a lesser degree than does total obstruction.[21] The rate at which the obstruction is produced may be responsible for this difference.[22]

Traditionally, the increased susceptibility to infection in obstructive uropathy has been attributed to "stasis." It is clear that urinary obstruction allows bacteria to multiply more readily in the *renal parenchyma*. Furthermore, the obstructed urine undoubtedly serves to transmit infection from one part of the kidney to the other. However, bacterial multiplica-

tion *in the urine* is not needed to initiate pyelonephritis when conditions of obstruction are present.[22]

Intrarenal Urinary Obstruction—Any damage to the kidney is likely to result in scarring of the tissue with obstruction of nephrons. The effect of such obstruction on susceptibility to infection depends on its location. In animals, scars in the renal cortex caused no increase in susceptibility, whereas scars in the renal papilla produced a dramatic rise.[23] This observation prompted tests to determine the lowest number of bacteria necessary for infection in different zones of the kidney. In the rabbit, at least 100,000 bacteria (*Esch. coli*) were needed to infect the cortex, whereas fewer than ten could produce infection in the medulla (Figure 10).[20] Because of such marked susceptibility to infection, the medulla and papilla were found to be the sites in the kidney where bacterial multiplication begins.[20] Of course, with obstruction of the medullary portion of the nephron, infection quickly spreads to the cortical nephrons which drain into the same collecting duct. Since the cortical extension of a medullary or papillary lesion invariably

Figure 10. Relative susceptibility of cortex and medulla to experimental infection.

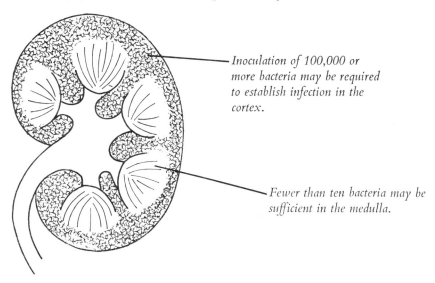

Inoculation of 100,000 or more bacteria may be required to establish infection in the cortex.

Fewer than ten bacteria may be sufficient in the medulla.

occupies a much larger area on the surface of the kidney, it is not surprising that the cortical spread of infection has always attracted attention. The evidence seems convincing, however, that the medulla and papilla are the sites where the decisive struggle determining whether or not infection supervenes in the kidney parenchyma takes place.[1] Consequently, one must look to the renal papilla and medulla to understand the pathogenesis of pyelonephritis.

The Medulla and Papilla—The conditions in the medullary and papillary zones of the kidney which may influence the fate of bacteria deposited there have received a great deal of attention. However, the situation is extraordinarily complex; in the peculiar physiological environment of the medulla and papilla are some factors which favor the survival of bacteria and others which adversely influence bacterial multiplication.[1] Some of these factors act directly on the

bacteria and others on host defense mechanisms. To complicate the situation further, changes in the physiological environment of the medulla and the renal papilla have a given effect on multiplication of bacteria present there and an opposite effect on multiplication of those bacteria in the urine and the lower urinary tract.[24-26]

For example, acidification of the urine by ingestion of such agents as methionine or ascorbic acid in suitable amounts has proved to be of benefit in the management of patients with chronic bacteriuria. When the pH of the urine is about 5, bacterial multiplication is hampered, and, although this does not cure the infection, it sometimes gives symptomatic relief.[27]

On the other hand, administering acidifying agents to rats causes an increase in their susceptibility to pyelonephritis. Acidification stimulates the formation of ammonia, which, in turn, inactivates the fourth component of complement. Complement is necessary for the integrity of antigen-antibody bactericidal systems in serum and for efficient phagocytosis. Thus, interference with these mechanisms tends to favor bacterial multiplication. Although the precise details of the phenomenon are not available, it can explain susceptibility to infection on a biochemical basis.[28]

A further example is water diuresis, which has been part of the traditional therapeutic regimen in patients with urinary tract infection. Only recently have attempts been made to find experimental and theoretical bases for its use. It is known that bacteria are transformed in vivo into atypical variants—i.e., spheroplasts or L-phase bacteria—by the action of certain antibiotics and serum antibody-complement-dependent systems.[29] Since the cell wall is modified or is totally lacking in L-phase bacteria, the cells are unprotected and may be osmotically sensitive. Thus, it has been found that lysis may occur in isotonic body fluids, because water passes into the L-phase cell. This does not occur in hypertonic fluids. Inasmuch as most of the medulla and the papillary region are hypertonic, they are presumably favorable to L-phase bacteria. It may be anticipated, then, that reducing the osmolarity of these zones by water diuresis greatly reduces the chance for survival of L-phase bacteria.

Water diuresis also increases the rate of blood flow in the medulla and papilla (where it is normally low) and thereby increases the availability of white cells at the inflammatory focus.[25]

Finally, high osmolarity, due to high salt and urea concentrations, interferes with the action of complement and the migration and function of polymorphonuclear leukocytes; therefore, by lowering the osmotic pressure, water diuresis should enhance the efficacy of the host defense mechanisms.

Partial support for these speculations comes from studies in animals which show that hematogenous pyelonephritis tends to be cured or prevented by chronic water diuresis.[24,25] However, not all animal studies are in agreement. In rats with Esch. coli bacteriuria, water diuresis is believed to impair bladder defense mechanisms and to interfere with clearance of bacteria.[9] Water diuresis in mice with bacteriuria leads to development of severe pyelonephritis and papillary necrosis.[26]

Some, but not all, experimental observations in animals and certain theoretical considerations suggest that water diuresis may benefit patients with pyelonephritis. Unfortunately, clinical evidence that this is the case is lacking. In addition, antibiotic therapy may be hampered if the antibiotic is greatly diluted by the large volume of urine during water diuresis.

SIGNIFICANCE OF DISEASES OF THE MEDULLA AND PAPILLA

With experimental evidence establishing the unique role of the renal medulla and papilla in the pathogenesis of pyelonephritis, there has been increasing recognition and appreciation of the clinical disorders of these zones of the kidney.

Renal Function in Pyelonephritis—The major renal functional changes in pyelonephritis are those caused by nephron loss. Damage may occur in any portion of the nephron. However, tubular structures are usually affected to the greatest extent because bacterial proliferation begins in the medulla. Intact glomeruli surrounded by damaged tissue are often seen in sections of the kidney in acute pyelonephritis (Figure 11). In addition to nephrons which are actually damaged by the infection, there are others

Figure 11. Section showing intact glomerulus surrounded by inflamed tissue.

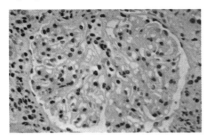

which are rendered nonfunctional. Thus, damaged and occluded medullary nephrons prevent the cortical nephrons (which share a collecting duct with them) from functioning effectively.

Since the cortical portion of the kidney is considerably larger than the medulla, an infection of similar extent would affect medullary functions proportionately more than cortical activities. Consequently, patients with pyelonephritis are more likely to have disturbances in medullary renal functions (urinary concentration, acid excretion, sodium reabsorption) than are patients with glomerular (cortical) renal disease.[30] For a discussion of renal functions, see Chapter 6.

Drugs, Alcohol, and Age—Ingestion of excessive quantities of analgesic mixtures containing phenacetin, aspirin, and often codeine has been clearly associated with papillary necrosis, interstitial nephritis, and the slower-developing but more insidious scarring called "papillary sclerosis."[1,31] When any of these disorders occurs in the presence of urinary infection, the effect on renal function may be catastrophic.

Papillary sclerosis and necrosis are found also in sickle-cell disease and chronic alcoholism and increase in frequency with aging. Some of these patients may also be taking large quantities of certain analgesics.[32-34]

Appreciation of the dangers of analgesic ingestion is important clinically, since discontinuation of the drugs along with treatment of the infection, if present, will probably arrest the progress of the disease. Patients are often reluctant to admit to excessive use of analgesics and must be questioned carefully.

Diabetes and Extrarenal Obstruction—Diabetes mellitus has long been known to predispose to papillary necrosis, presumably because of vascular narrowing in the kidney. Extrarenal urinary obstruction regularly produces papillary necrosis in animals, and the association has been noted in man. However, some authors have pointed out that the tissue sloughed by the necrosis may get stuck in the ureter and so cause the obstruction. Such a possibility is difficult to rule out.[35]

Papillary necrosis is diagnosed by the finding of the sloughed necrotic papillary tissue in the urine or by characteristic changes revealed by pyelography.[36] Sometimes, however, the x-ray changes are not diagnostic, and the renal lesions cause rapid shrinkage of all or part of the kidney, as occurs in pyelonephritis.

Considerable experimental work and clinical observation in the past few years have added immeasurably to our knowledge of the pathogenesis of pyelonephritis, and a great deal of this information can be translated into concepts useful for patient management. As important as any other aspect of the work of recent years has been the recognition that so much of what we thought we knew up to about ten years ago is incorrect. Only by continued study in the clinic and in the laboratory will we fill the gaps in our knowledge and thereby improve the treatment of patients.

BIBLIOGRAPHY

1. Freedman, L. R.: Pyelonephritis and Urinary Tract Infection, in Diseases of the Kidney (edited by M. B. Strauss and L. G. Welt), p. 469. Boston: Little, Brown & Company, 1963.

2. Kunin, C. M., Deutscher, R., and Paquin, A., Jr.: Urinary Tract Infection in School Children: An Epidemiologic, Clinical and Laboratory Study, Medicine, 43:91, 1964.

3. Norden, C. W., and Kass, E. H.: Bacteriuria of Pregnancy—A Critical Appraisal, Ann. Rev. Med., 19: 431, 1968.

4. Stamey, T. A., Govan, D. E., and Palmer, J. M.: The Localization and Treatment of Urinary Tract Infections: The Role of Bactericidal Urine Levels as Opposed to Serum Levels, Medicine, 44:1, 1965.

5. Beeson, P. B.: The Case against the Catheter, Am. J. Med., 24:1, 1958.

6. Meares, E. M., and Stamey, T. A.: Bacteriologic Localization Patterns in Bacterial Prostatitis and Urethritis, Invest. Urol., 5:492, 1968.

7. Norden, C. W., Green, G. M., and Kass, E. H.: Antibacterial Mechanisms of the Urinary Bladder, J. Clin. Invest., 47:2689, 1968.

8. Cobbs, C. G., and Kaye, D.: Antibacterial Mechanisms in the Urinary Bladder, Yale J. Biol. & Med., 40:93, 1967.

9. Freedman, L. R.: Experimental Pyelonephritis. XIII. On the Ability of Water Diuresis to Induce Susceptibility to E. Coli Bacteriuria in the Normal Rat, Yale J. Biol. & Med., 39:255, 1967.

10. Michie, A. J.: Chronic Pyelonephritis Mimicking Ureteral Obstructions, Pediat. Clin. North America, 6:1117, 1959.

11. Glenn, J. F. (Editor): Workshop in Ureteral Reflux in Children. Washington: National Academy of Sciences/National Research Council, 1966.

12. Miall, W. E., Kass, E. H., Ling, J., and Stuart, K. L.: Factors Influencing Arterial Pressure in the General Population in Jamaica, Brit. M. J., 2:497, 1962.

13. Freedman, L. R., Phair, J. P., Seki, M., Hamilton, H. B., and Nefzger, M. D.: The Epidemiology of Urinary Tract Infections in Hiroshima, Yale J. Biol. & Med., 37:262, 1965.

14. Kunin, C. M., and McCormack, R. C.: An Epidemiologic Study of Bacteriuria and Blood Pressure among Nuns and Working Women, New England J. Med., 278:635, 1968.

15. Bricker, N. S.: Obstructive Nephropathy, in Diseases of the Kidney (edited by M. B. Strauss and L. G. Welt), p. 728. Boston: Little, Brown & Company, 1963.

16. Drachman, R. H., Root, R. K., and Wood, W. B., Jr.: Studies on the Effect of Experimental Nonketotic Diabetes Mellitus on Antibacterial Defense. I. Demonstration of a Defect in Phagocytosis, J. Exper. Med., 124:227, 1966.

17. Pometta, D., Rees, S. B., Younger, D., and Kass, E. H.: Asymptomatic Bacteriuria in Diabetes Mellitus, New England J. Med., 276:1118, 1967.

18. Heptinstall, R. H.: The Limitations of the Pathological Diagnosis of Chronic Pyelonephritis, in Renal Disease, Ed. 2 (edited by D. A. K. Black), p. 350. Oxford: Blackwell Scientific Publications, 1967.

19. Guze, L. B., and Beeson, P. B.: Experimental Pyelonephritis. I. Effect of Ureteral Ligation on the Course of Bacterial Infection in the Kidney of the Rat, J. Exper. Med., 104:803, 1956.

20. Freedman, L. R., and Beeson, P. B.: Experimental Pyelonephritis. IV. Observations on Infections Resulting from Direct Inoculation of Bacteria in Different Zones of the Kidney, Yale J. Biol. & Med., 30:406, 1958.

21. Guze, L. B., Hubert, E., and Kalmanson, G. M.: Pyelonephritis. VI. Observations of the Effects of Congenital, Partial Ureteral Obstruction on Susceptibility of the Rat Kidney to Infection, J. Infect. Dis., 115:500, 1965.

22. Freedman, L. R., Kaminskas, E., and Beeson, P. B.: Experimental Pyelonephritis. VII. Evidence on the Mechanisms by Which Obstruction of Urine Flow Enhances Susceptibility to Pyelonephritis, Yale J. Biol. & Med., 33:65, 1960.

23. Rocha, H., Guze, L. B., Freedman, L. R., and Beeson, P. B.: Experimental Pyelonephritis. III. The Influence of Localized Injury in Different Parts of the Kidney on Susceptibility to Bacillary Infection, Yale J. Biol. & Med., 30:341, 1958.

24. Andriole, V. T., and Epstein, F. H.: Prevention of Pyelonephritis by Water Diuresis: Evidence for the Role of Medullary Hypertonicity in Promoting Renal Infection, J. Clin. Invest., 44:73, 1965.

25. Andriole, V. T.: Acceleration of the Inflammatory Response of the Renal Medulla by Water Diuresis, J. Clin. Invest., 45:847, 1966.

26. Keane, W. F., and Freedman, L. R.: Experimental Pyelonephritis. XIV. Pyelonephritis in Normal Mice Produced by Inoculation of E. Coli into the Bladder Lumen during Water Diuresis, Yale J. Biol. & Med., 40:231, 1967.

27. Bodel, P. T., Cotran, R., and Kass, E. H.: Cranberry Juice and the Antibacterial Action of Hippuric Acid, J. Lab. & Clin. Med., 54:881, 1959.

28. Freedman, L. R., and Beeson, P. B.: Experimental Pyelonephritis. VIII. The Effect of Acidifying Agents on Susceptibility to Infection, Yale J. Biol. & Med., 33:318, 1961.

29. Guze, L. B. (Editor): Microbial Protoplasts, Spheroplasts and L-Forms. Baltimore: The Williams & Wilkins Company, 1968.

30. Beck, D., Freedman, L. R., Levitin, H., Ferris, T. F., and Epstein, F. H.: Effect of Experimental Pyelonephritis on the Renal Concentrating Ability of the Rat, Yale J. Biol. & Med., *34:*52, 1961.

31. Fellner, S. K., and Tuttle, E. P.: The Clinical Syndrome of Analgesic Abuse, Arch. Int. Med., *124:*379, 1969.

32. Mostofi, F. K., Vorder Bruegge, C. F., and Diggs, L. W.: Lesions in Kidneys Removed for Unilateral Hematuria in Sickle-Cell Disease, A.M.A. Arch. Path., *63:*336, 1957.

33. Edmondson, H. A., Reynolds, T. B., and Jacobson, H. G.: Renal Papillary Necrosis with Special Reference to Chronic Alcoholism; A Report of 20 Cases, Arch. Int. Med., *118:*255, 1966.

34. Keresztury, S., and Megyeri, L.: Histology of Renal Pyramids with Special Regard to Changes Due to Ageing, Acta Morph. Acad. Sci. Hung., *11:*205, 1962.

35. Harrow, B. R.: Renal Papillary Necrosis: A Critique of Pathogenesis, J. Urol., *97:*203, 1967.

36. Bengtsson, U.: A Comparative Study of Chronic Non-Obstructive Pyelonephritis and Renal Papillary Necrosis, Acta med. scandinav., *172* (Supplement 388): 1962.

GENERAL REFERENCES

Beeson, P. B.: Urinary Tract Infection and Pyelonephritis, in Renal Disease, Ed. 2 (edited by D. A. K. Black), p. 382. Oxford: Blackwell Scientific Publications, 1967.

Kimmelstiel, P.: Asymptomatic Bacteriuria, a Hypothetical Concept, Should Be Treated with Caution, in Controversy in Internal Medicine (edited by F. J. Ingelfinger, A. S. Relman, and M. Finland), p. 313. Philadelphia: W. B. Saunders Company, 1966.

Kleeman, C. R., Hewitt, W. L., and Guze, L. B.: Pyelonephritis, Medicine, *39:*3, 1960.

Kunin, C. M.: Asymptomatic Bacteriuria, Ann. Rev. Med., *17:*383, 1966.

Pawlowski, J. M., Bloxdorf, J. W., and Kimmelstiel, P.: Chronic Pyelonephritis; A Morphologic and Bacteriologic Study, New England J. Med., *268:*965, 1963.

Sanford, J. P., and Barnett, J. A.: Immunologic Responses in Urinary-Tract Infections, J.A.M.A., *192:*587, 1965.

Savage, W. E., Hajj, S. N., and Kass, E. H.: Demographic and Prognostic Characteristics of Bacteriuria in Pregnancy, Medicine, *46:*385, 1967.

Stamey, T. A., Fair, W. R., Timothy, M. M., and Chung, H. K.: Antibacterial Nature of Prostatic Fluid, Nature, London, *218:*444, 1968.

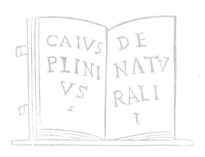

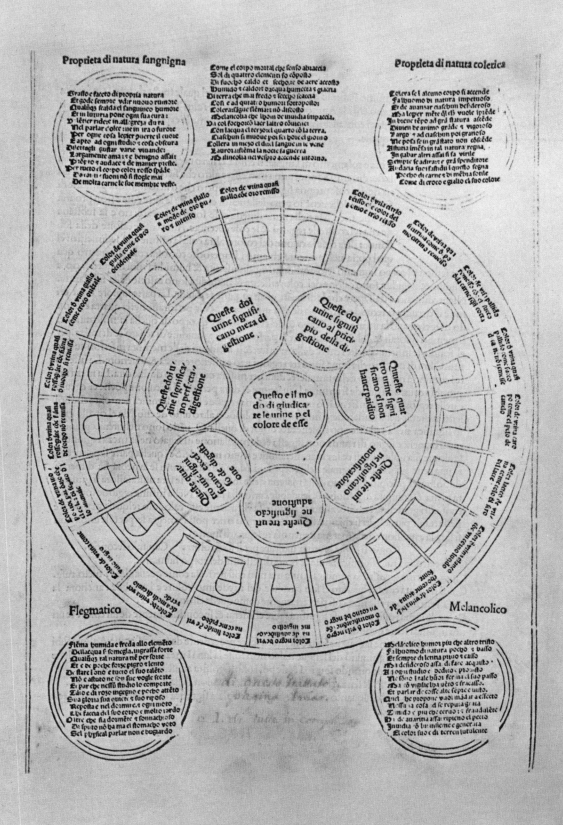

3
Technics of Laboratory Diagnosis

The presence of infection in any part of the urinary system usually produces significant changes in the urine. These changes can be detected and evaluated by the methods of quantitative bacteriology and by routine procedures of urinalysis. In addition, the patient may be examined by one or more radiologic technics to help establish a diagnosis.

QUANTITATIVE BACTERIOLOGY OF URINE

Significant Bacteriuria—The concept of significant bacteriuria was introduced to distinguish between urinary contaminants and organisms actually multiplying in the kidneys, ureters, and bladder.[1] Culture of a properly collected, cleanly voided midstream sample in health is sterile or contains 1,000 or fewer organisms per ml. of urine due to the normal urethral flora. In contrast, Kass found 100,000 or more organisms per ml.

of urine in 95 percent of cases of clinical pyelonephritis.[2] He therefore selected this number as evidence of significant bacteriuria. In actual fact, when an infection exists, usually more than 1,000,000 organisms per ml. of urine are cultured.

Surveys of various presumably healthy populations by Kass[2] and others,[3,4] in which the methods of quantitative bacteriology on cleanly voided midstream urine were used, indicate that most individuals with significant bacteriuria are asymptomatic, as are most with chronic infections of the renal parenchyma prior to the final phase of their illness.

Routine bacteriologic study of urine is readily performed in most physicians' offices with the "secretary-nurse-laboratory technician" trained to carry out the essential operations of collecting the sample and preparing cultures and stained specimens.

Collection of Specimen—To be of value in diagnosis, bacteriologic analysis must be done on urine that contains a representative sample of urinary tract flora. Contamination of the specimen by bacteria commonly present in the urethra, on the external genitalia, and on the perineum must be avoided. The technic used to obtain urine suitable for bacteriologic analysis depends on the sex of the patient.

In men, the glans penis is carefully cleansed with soap, water, and sterile sponges. Then, during forceful urination, the urine stream is caught consecutively in three sterile disposable clear plastic cups, and immediately each is covered with a tightly fitting lid.

In women, additional precautions are required. The collection can be made on the toilet, over a washbowl, or on a special urologic examining table. The following instructions, printed on a card given to the patient, have been helpful[5]:

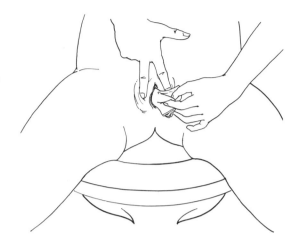

Figure 12. Collection of urine sample from women. With the labia held apart, washing is done from high up front toward the back with gauze soaked in soap.

Cleanliness in the collection of your urine specimen will make it possible for us to give you better care. Please follow the instructions carefully in the order they are given.

1. Remove your underpants.

2. Wash your hands carefully. To do this, you must soap them thoroughly, then rinse, and shake off excess water.

3. Take one wet gauze sponge from the bowl of sponges soaking in green soap.

4. Spread yourself with the other hand and wash with the wet gauze. Do this well, from high up front toward the back (Figure 12). When finished, drop the used gauze into the waste container.

5. Continue to keep yourself spread and wash yourself the same way with a second wet sponge, then with a third, a fourth, and a fifth, and discard each sponge as you finish with it.

6. Remain spread and start urinating. Once you have started, catch some urine in a sterile disposable clear plastic cup which is held so that it does not touch your skin or clothing (Figure 12a).

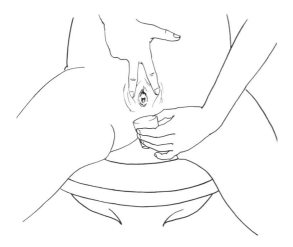

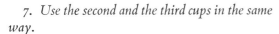

Figure 12a. The cup is held so that it does not touch the body, and a sample is obtained only while the subject is urinating with the labia held apart.

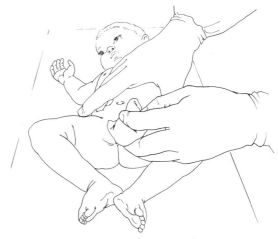

Figure 13. The Perez reflex to induce urination in an infant. The infant's external genitalia are first washed thoroughly.

7. *Use the second and the third cups in the same way.*

8. *Cover the cups and notify attendant.*

The first specimen is considered to be representative of urine from the anterior urethra and its appendages, such as the prostate in the male. It should be examined by naked eye—as should the other two specimens—for evidence of gross abnormality, such as blood, blood clots, shreds of pus, etc., and should be cultured if infection of the urethra and its appendages is suspected. The second, or midstream, specimen collected is considered representative of bladder urine and is used for bacteriologic examination and sensitivity studies, whether or not it is normal in appearance. The third specimen is said to reflect disease in the upper urinary tract, but such a statement is probably erroneous. This specimen may be used for urinalysis.

Other methods of urine collection are necessary with certain patients. In infants or very young children, the penis or female puden-

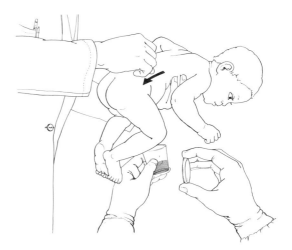

Figure 13a. Stroking of the paraspinal muscles elicits the Perez reflex and results in urination.

dum is cleansed as described for adults. While the infant is held face down over a sterile container, urination can be stimulated by pressure over the suprapubic area or by firm stroking of the paraspinal muscles to elicit the Perez reflex (Figures 13 and 13a). This

Figure 14. Position of infant during catheterization.

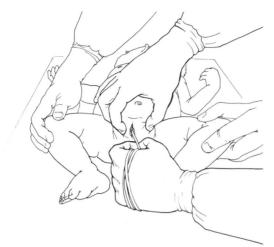

results in crying, extension of the back, re-flexion of the legs and arms, and urination. A sterile plastic urine-collecting bag can also be used. It is put on after the genitalia have been cleaned as described and is held in place by a tightly pinned diaper. The bag must be removed as soon as the infant voids. If no

urine appears in forty-five minutes, cleansing must be repeated and a new bag applied.

It is difficult to avoid contamination of the urine collected from infants even though all possible precautions are taken. Catheterization may be necessary (Figure 14), or, as pre-ferred by some pediatric nephrologists, urine may be collected for culture with a sterile percutaneous bladder tap (Figures 15 and 15a). In infants, however, proper use of this technic requires skill and practice.

When patients are bedfast, urine can be collected while they are sitting on a bedside commode. Under some conditions—uncon-sciousness, un-co-operativeness, after deliv-ery, etc.—catheterization may be necessary. However, to avoid catheterization when it is difficult to collect a cleanly voided sample, some physicians and pediatricians use aseptic percutaneous needle puncture of the blad-der.[6,7] Since the procedure is considered safe and is painless when properly done, it is used routinely in some hospitals to collect urine

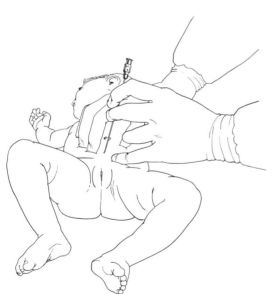

Figure 15. Percutaneous bladder tap. The needle in position before insertion.

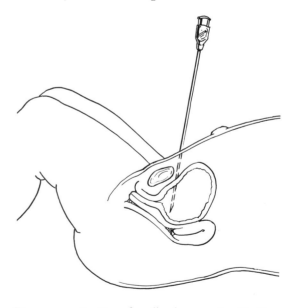

Figure 15a. Position of needle after entry into bladder.

for culture. A few red cells may appear in the urinary sediment although none are seen in the voided sample. Complications are rare; none occurred in 3,000 taps done at Stanford University.[8]

Microscopy—By examining gram-stained *uncentrifuged* urine, the technician can confirm the presence of bacteria and quickly make a useful estimation of their number (Figure 16). If a single organism is seen in each high-power field, a presumptive diagnosis of significant bacteriuria is justified, and therapy may be started before the results of cultures are available, as discussed below.

The search for bacteria and a count can be done on the *unstained* and *centrifuged* urinary sediment.[9] For this purpose, the phase-contrast microscope is best.[10] With this instrument, bacteria are more easily recognized and distinguished from debris than with the standard light microscope (Figures 16a and 16b). If more than twenty organisms per high-power field are seen, the diagnosis of significant bacteriuria is positive.

An advantage of the microscopic search is that bacteriuria can be detected immediately and treatment begun without delay if the physician deems it necessary. In the meantime, urine cultures are prepared and sensitivity tests are run so that a more appropriate antibiotic can be prescribed if needed. While the results of the cultures are pending, the patient's response to the initial treatment can be assessed by examination of the urine for bacteria. If treatment has been successful, bacteria will disappear from the urinary tract within twenty-four to forty-eight hours, and none will be seen under the microscope.

Culture—Urine specimens must be cultured within thirty minutes of collection or be refrigerated immediately. They can be stored for as long as forty-eight hours at 8°C. without significant growth of bacteria.

Urine may be cultured in an agar pour plate and an estimate of the number of bacteria made by colony count. It may be streaked on the surface of an agar plate and the colonies counted if a calibrated loop is used to make the streak. Generally, urine is streaked on blood agar to give a total bac-

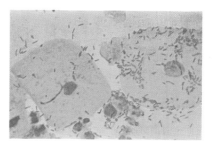

Figure 16. *Gram stain of uncentrifuged urine (standard light microscope).*

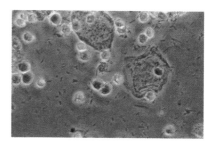

Figure 16a. *Unstained centrifuged urine (phase-contrast microscope).*

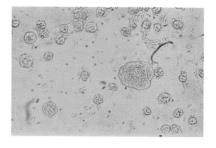

Figure 16b. *Unstained centrifuged urine (standard light microscope).*

terial count and on highly selective media to indicate gram-negative rods (Figures 17 and 17a). Simple and ingenious inexpensive culture devices[11] are becoming commercially available and will soon make quantitative urine cultures a routine office procedure.

With one properly obtained urine sample, the distinction between bacteria responsible for infection and contaminants can be made correctly in eight out of ten cases, i.e., with a confidence limit of 80 percent. If two samples are used, the confidence limit increases to 95 percent.[12,13] Contamination should be suspected if replicate cultures or cultures made at different times do not agree in either number or type of organism, if two or more organisms are isolated in large numbers, or if diphtheroids, *Staphylococcus* sp., or microaerophilic streptococci are predominant. (It should be recalled that in 80 percent or more of uncomplicated urinary tract infections, *Esch. coli* is the causative organism; in complicated cases, one or more species of *Proteus, Enterobacter,* or *Pseudomonas* and, rarely, *Staph. aureus* and certain other organisms are more likely to be encountered.)

On the other hand, if symptoms and signs continue unabated or if cultures are sterile (even though leukocytes are present in the urinary sediment), the infection may be due to *Mycobacterium tuberculosis* or to an anaerobic organism which must be cultured by appropriate methods.

Infection without Bacteriuria—Infection may exist in the urinary tract without producing bacteriuria. This may occur when there is an obstruction below the infected site. It may also be due to perinephric abscesses, hematogenous staphylococcus pyelonephritis, or so-called "burned-out" chronic pyelonephritis.

Other Tests for Bacteriuria—Chemical and enzymatic tests for bacteriuria have been devised and depend on the presence of bacterial

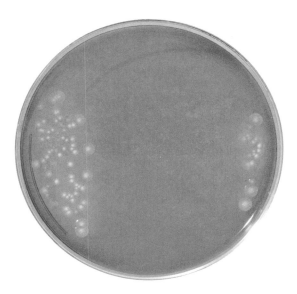

Figure 17. Blood agar streak plate of appropriately diluted urine indicates total bacterial count.

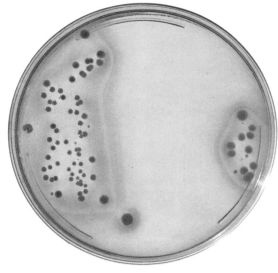

Figure 17a. Growth on the selective MacConkey agar streak plate indicates gram-negative organisms.

metabolites or certain enzymes in greater amounts than normal in the urine.[14-16] Measurement of urine enzyme activities by tetrazolium reductase or glucose oxidase tests, for instance, does not as yet distinguish between damage due to infection and that caused by other means. These (and similar methods) are potentially powerful tools but must be developed further before they become useful.

URINALYSIS

Infection in the urinary system evokes a wide variety of reactions which depend on its locality, activity, and severity.[17] In asymptomatic bacteriuria, the urine may not be abnormal in any respect except that the specific gravity may be rather low in pregnant patients. In acute pyelonephritis, the urine usually contains a small amount of protein—0.5 to 1 Gm.—in a twenty-four-hour specimen, many white cells (both singly and in clumps), a few red cells, and, characteristically, many white-cell casts. In chronic pyelonephritis, the urine is usually pale and the specific gravity low; there is an insignificant proteinuria —0.5 to 1 Gm. in twenty-four hours; and there is a paucity of renal epithelial cells and casts in the sediment. In complicated chronic infections of the lower urinary tract, the urine is usually cloudy, "thick," and filled with shreds of tissue, pus, and blood clots.

The early-morning specimen is concentrated and therefore more likely to reveal abnormalities than a specimen obtained at some other time. It is usually satisfactory for routine examination. However, analysis of properly preserved twenty-four-hour samples gives a more accurate quantitative measurement of protein and other constituents than does the random specimen. In females, it may be necessary to pack the vagina to avoid contamination of the urine with vaginal epithelial cells, white cells, and white-cell clumps if a discharge is present. The urine should be examined within thirty minutes after it is passed or be stored under refrigeration.

Color—Infection has no effect on the color of the urine. However, its presence may produce a hazy or cloudy urine; or the urine may be "thick" or filled with shreds of mucus and pus. Rarely, blood and clots may tinge it red, or it may contain renal papillary tissue.

Odor—Fresh urine has an aromatic odor. Urine allowed to stand at room temperature soon acquires a characteristic pungency owing to ammonia formed by bacterial action. For the same reason, the urine tends to be ammoniacal during infection. In severe infection, it may have a particularly unpleasant fishy odor.

Specific Gravity, Osmolality, and Refractive Index—These properties are related to one another because all reflect the quantity of dissolved solids in the urine.[18] The most important urinary solutes are urea and sodium chloride.

Commonly, an inexpensive hydrometer is used to measure specific gravity, but often this instrument is inaccurate. Osmolality is determined accurately by freezing-point depression. (For a discussion of osmolality, see Box 7, page 103.) The expense of the instrument—the cryostat—and the time required for the determination make this technic impractical for the physician's office. The estimation of refractive index is a relatively simple and rapid procedure that can be done with a clinical hand refractometer. The refractometer technic is particularly useful inasmuch as the determination requires only a single drop of urine. Refractometer readings are easily translated into specific gravity or osmolality by means of conversion tables or charts.

The specific gravity of protein-free serum (and thus of the glomerular filtrate) is about 1.007.* During the passage of this filtrate through the tubules and collecting ducts, the specific gravity is altered by tubular reabsorption or secretion of water and solutes. Thus, in the patient on a normal diet, inability to concentrate the urine nearly always indicates disease of the kidney.

Infection may prevent adequate concentration of urine. Kaitz[19] has shown that pregnant patients with asymptomatic bacteriuria who are unable to concentrate the urine adequately regain this ability after treatment with appropriate antibiotics. This observation lends support to the concept that some cases of significant asymptomatic bacteriuria may involve the kidneys.

Failure to concentrate the urine is typical of chronic pyelonephritis. In fact, it occurs in any disease that involves the medulla and that produces chronic renal medullary failure —for example, severe potassium deficiency, hypercalcemia, gout, congenital renal disease (especially polycystic disease), analgesic abuse, chronic lead poisoning, and various forms of ischemia. In all these diseases, the cortex and glomeruli are affected only after extensive medullary damage. On the other hand, in primary glomerular diseases, such as glomerulonephritis and diabetes, the ability to concentrate properly does not diminish until late, when the medulla is finally affected.

Loss of concentrating ability also occurs when there are intrinsic renal tubular defects, e.g., in nephrogenic diabetes insipidus. Furthermore, patients with diabetes insipidus

and those who have compulsive-water-drinking syndromes are unable to concentrate their urine up to 1.010.

If a single specimen of urine, such as that first passed in the morning, has a specific gravity exceeding 1.020, it is usually unnecessary to run a specific-gravity concentration test. However, if this test is to be attempted, the physician must remember that the kidneys will be unable to concentrate to high levels unless adequate amounts of solutes are being consumed by the patient or are being produced by catabolism. For this reason, difficulties may arise in patients on low-sodium or protein-deficient diets. In addition, during spontaneous or induced diuresis, the urine specific gravity will remain low, and the patient will be unable to concentrate. (For a discussion of the concentrating and diluting mechanism, see page 103.)

Unfortunately, the concentration test cannot be used to differentiate between severe chronic infection of the kidney and severe chronic glomerulonephritis. One might speculate that creatinine clearance in chronic infections of the kidney should be normal or nearly normal and concentrating ability greatly diminished or virtually lacking. (The clearance concept is discussed on page 95.) Conversely, in glomerulonephritis, creatinine clearance should be low, and concentrating ability should be normal. However, actual observation does not agree with this speculation.[20] It is generally agreed that surviving nephrons hypertrophy and take over major functional activity of the end-stage kidney. In the surviving nephrons, the loss of glomerular function and the loss of concentrating ability are not equally reduced. End-stage kidneys are prone to lose salt as a result of disproportionate hypertrophy of the proximal portions of the surviving nephrons.[21]

---

*A urine with specific gravity greater than 1.010 indicates that concentration has occurred, whereas a specific gravity less than 1.010 denotes dilution. The term *isosthenuria* is used to describe urine having a specific gravity that is consistently 1.010. In *hyposthenuria*, the specific gravity of the urine is less than 1.008.

Hydrogen-Ion Concentration—The pH of the urine varies throughout the day. Usually, urine is acid because of acidic metabolites produced by normal breakdown of body tissues and nutrients. It becomes less acid after meals. In urinary tract infections, the urine may be alkaline mainly because of ammonia produced by bacterial decomposition of urea. For example, in *Proteus* infections, the urine is consistently at about pH 8 or higher. On the other hand, tuberculous infection of the kidney is commonly associated with a consistently acid urine. Determination of pH should always be done on freshly voided urine, or special precautions should be taken to avoid erroneous results that could be caused by bacterial growth.

Proteinuria—In health, the urine contains small amounts of protein consisting of albumin and various globulins which are derived from plasma.[22,23] In addition, it contains proteins secreted by the kidney tubules, by the remainder of the urinary tract, and, in males, by the prostate.

In healthy adults, the twenty-four-hour excretion is generally less than 250 mg. and is not detected by the usual tests for proteinuria.

Fixed and reproducible proteinuria means renal disease, and its cause should be thoroughly investigated. Usually, in bacterial infections of the urinary tract, the proteinuria is negligible to moderate in amount; that is, the twenty-four-hour excretion does not exceed 1 Gm. In chronic pyelonephritis with marked and progressive renal involvement, proteinuria may be minimal or absent. Transitory proteinuria may be associated with severe anemia, congestive cardiac failure, central-nervous-system lesions, thyroid disorders, and most acute diseases, especially if fever is present.

Many observers think that, in renal disease,

Figure 18. Appearance of results in some protein tests.

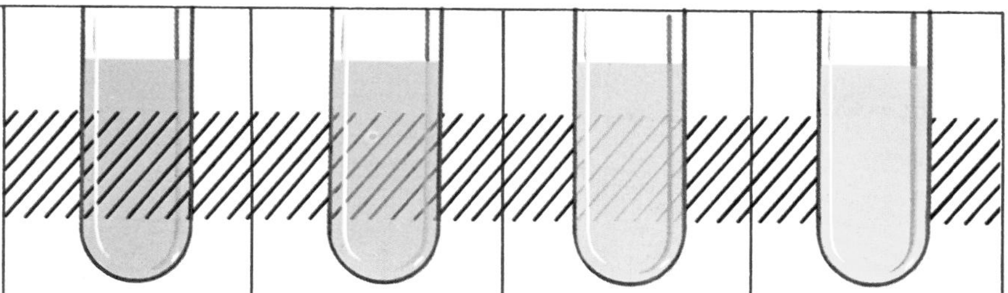

TESTS 1. Heat and acetic acid *or* 2. Sulfosalicylic acid	No turbidity Black lines clearly visible	Slight turbidity Black lines clearly visible	Moderate turbidity Black lines still visible	White cloud Black lines not visible
3. Albustix®				
4. Combistix®				
Report results as	0 Nil	1+ Trace	1+ to 2+ Intermediate	3+ to 4+ Heavy
Results indicate approximate range of protein	0	<30 mg./100 ml.	30-100 mg./100 ml.	>100 mg./100 ml.

Table 1

CAUSES OF FALSE REACTIONS IN SOME PROTEIN TESTS[17]

Conditions	Methods		
	Heat and Acetic Acid	Sulfosalicylic Acid	Albustix or Combistix
Highly buffered alkaline urine	False negative	False negative	False positive
p-Aminosalicylic acid in urine with preservatives	False positive	False positive	No effect
X-ray contrast media	False positive	False positive	No effect
Penicillin in high concentration	False positive	False positive	No effect
Sulfisoxazole metabolites	No effect	False positive	No effect
Tolbutamide metabolites	False positive	False positive	No effect

protein reaches the urinary tract by penetrating abnormal glomerular capillary walls. This appears to be the source of most urinary protein. Nevertheless, proteinuria may develop if tubular reabsorption of proteins is not normal. In addition, plasma proteins may be secreted into the tubules and, via the lymphatic system, into the renal pelvis. The genito-urinary tract is also a source of urinary protein. Combinations of these sources may occur during abnormal protein excretion.

Three clinical tests for proteinuria are commonly used. The appearance of the results obtained with these tests at various concentration ranges of protein is compared in Figure 18. Usual causes of false-positive reactions are given in Table 1.

Quantitative determinations of urinary protein are done preferably on a twenty-four-hour sample. The biuret test is probably the simplest and generally most satisfactory. However, the standard of reference is the Kjeldahl method for nitrogen determination.

Quantitative data are valuable in establishing a diagnosis and also in following the course of renal disease. To make comparisons possible among infants, children, and adults, the calculations must take into account the size of the patient. This may be expressed in weight, height, or surface area. Since patients with renal disease are often edematous, both weight and surface area may change abruptly. For this reason, twenty-four-hour urine excretion of protein and other quantitative urine measurements are corrected by the cube of the patient's height. On this basis, normal adults excrete from 20 to 80 mg. of protein per twenty-four hours, with an arbitrary upper limit of 100 to 150 mg. Patients with urinary tract infection usually excrete either normal amounts or up to 1 Gm. per day.

A variety of technics, including electrophoresis and immunodiffusion, are available to separate urine proteins. In addition, methods have been developed to measure the renal clearances of the thirty serum proteins.[24] The protein-clearance data are valuable in diagnosing "lipoid nephrosis" from any cause. In this situation, there is a highly selective proteinuria consisting predominantly of serum proteins with small molecular weight. As yet, no specific protein or combination of proteins has been found to indicate the presence of infection. Similarly, no protein-clearance abnormalities have been correlated with any form of kidney or urinary tract infection.

Glucose and Other Reducing Substances—There are many reducing substances in the urine—for instance, glucose, fructose, galactose, pentose, homogentisic acid, and ascorbic acid. None of these is specifically related to infection, except that, in the diabetic patient, there is the well-known relationship between infection and the disease state. This is particularly evident with uncontrolled glycosuria. In addition to diabetes mellitus, inherited renal tubular defects or brain injury, excitement, or intravenous glucose infusions may induce glycosuria.

The determination of reducing substances, including glucose, by standard laboratory procedures depends on their ability to reduce copper solutions. If the exact nature of the reducing substance must be known, additional analytical methods are necessary. For this purpose, several systems of chromatography have been developed.

Various procedures have been devised to make measuring glucose in the urine both convenient and reasonably accurate. They require specially prepared test materials containing the enzyme glucose oxidase, and these are commercially available as Tes-Tape® (urine sugar analysis paper, Lilly) and Clini-

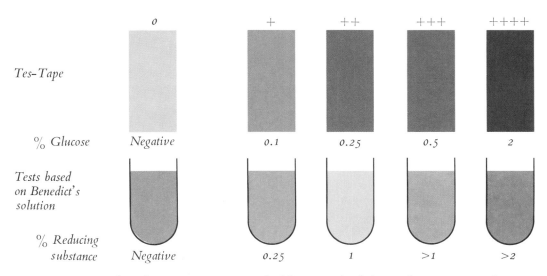

Figure 19. Appearance of results in an enzymatic method (Tes-Tape) of glucose determination and in tests based on Benedict's solution.

Table 2

THE EFFECTS OF SUBSTANCES FOUND IN URINE ON GLUCOSE TESTS[17]

Substance	Enzyme Tests*	Benedict's Solution
Galactose	No reaction	Positive
Lactose	No reaction	Positive
Fructose	No reaction	Positive
Pentose	No reaction	Positive
Creatinine	No reaction	False positive
Homogentisic acid	No reaction	False positive
Uric acid	No reaction	False positive
Salicylates	No reaction	False positive
Penicillin	No reaction	False positive†
Chloral hydrate	No reaction	False positive
Glucosamine	No reaction	False positive
Streptomycin	No reaction	False positive
Isoniazid	No reaction	False positive
p-Aminosalicylic acid	No reaction	False positive
Ascorbic acid	No reaction‡	False positive

*Either Tes-Tape or Clinistix.   ‡Large quantities may delay color development.
†When penicillin is present in large amounts.

stix®. Both tests reliably detect 0.1 percent or less of glucose and thus are more sensitive than tests based on copper reduction (Figure 19). Furthermore, because they depend on enzymatic action, they are specific for glucose (Table 2).

In some clinics, up to 20 percent of female patients with diabetes have significant bacteriuria, but only about 2 percent of these are found to have chronic pyelonephritis upon examination of kidneys at autopsy.[25] *This is an argument against the concept that all patients with significant bacteriuria will develop chronic kidney infections.* Nevertheless, diabetic patients require special care and should be examined very closely for evidence of urinary tract infection and for the presence of co-existing disorders, such as papillary necrosis.

Ketonuria—In healthy individuals, the ketone bodies—β-hydroxybutyric acid, acetoacetic acid, and acetone—are formed in the liver but are completely metabolized so that only occasionally do negligible amounts appear in the urine. Accumulation of these substances in urine occurs in any disorder of altered carbohydrate metabolism. They are found in uncontrolled diabetes, with starvation, vomiting, and dehydration, and following anesthesia, strenuous exercise, or exposure to severe cold. Accordingly, ketonuria may be present during urinary tract infections if carbohydrate metabolism is not normal.

Occult Blood—Many chemical tests have been devised to detect occult blood in the urine, but up to now none have been widely used in clinical practice. Unfortunately, none of the "dipstick" or "tablet" tests currently available can distinguish among hemoglobinuria, hematuria, and myoglobinuria. The pigments hemoglobin and myoglobin can be identified by either spectroscopic or immunologic methods. Gross hematuria is not commonly observed with acute infections of the kidney, although it may be present when the infection is located in the urinary tract. Microhematuria is a common finding in most acute urinary tract infections. It is also present in tuberculosis of the urinary tract and in bilharziasis (schistosomiasis).

Preparation of Sediment—Microscopic examination of urinary sediment should be done routinely. For this, a well-mixed fresh urine sample is needed. If the examination must be delayed for no more than an hour, the urine should be stored in a refrigerator, but, even then, a number of cells and casts may be destroyed during this time. Urine samples can be preserved by adding formalin or commercially available preservative tablets. However, since samples with preservative are not suitable for chemical analysis, a separate portion should be set aside for these tests.

If the sediment is particularly heavy, a drop of fresh uncentrifuged urine should be examined, for it may provide adequate evidence for diagnosis. Usually, however, centrifugation of the urine is necessary to obtain sufficient sediment for examination. If a routine procedure for concentrating and examining the sediment is followed closely at all times, comparison of results is possible with some degree of accuracy, both from day to day and from patient to patient. A satisfactory technic may be outlined as follows[26]:

1. Place 15 ml. of urine in a chemically clean conical tube and centrifuge at 2,000 r.p.m. for five minutes.

2. Remove the tube from the machine and quickly invert so that the supernate can be poured off. Immediately turn the tube upright, and suspend the button of sediment in the remaining urine by thorough mixing with a small glass rod.

3. With a fine pipette, transfer one drop of the suspension to an absolutely clean slide. If desired, the sediment may be stained with Brodie-Prescott,[27] Sternheimer-Malbin, or methylene blue. Cover the preparation, either stained or unstained, with a clean cover slip and examine while it is wet.

The time required for a thorough examination by an experienced person is five to ten minutes. A rough quantitation of the content can be made by counting the individual elements in ten or more high-power fields and expressing the result as an average. *The phase-contrast microscope is preferred for examination of urinary sediment.* If the standard bright-field microscope is used, the condenser should be racked down and the diaphragm closed so that the light is subdued; this makes recognition of the various elements somewhat more certain.

The Normal Sediment—In health, the urine contains small numbers of cells and other elements derived from the whole length of the genito-urinary tract—casts and epithelial cells from nephrons; epithelial cells from the pelves, ureters, bladder, urethra, and vagina; and mucous threads and spermatozoa. A few erythrocytes and leukocytes, apparently reaching the urine by diapedesis from any part of the urinary tract, also may be present.

Two to three red blood cells and four to five leukocytes per high-power field, with occasional hyaline and granular casts, are accepted as normal. Large numbers of erythrocytes, leukocytes, and casts may appear in the urine of healthy subjects after strenuous exercise or exposure to severe cold.

Significance of Casts—Casts are thought to be "moldings" of renal tubules. The principal sites of formation in disease are the distal convolutions of the tubules and the collecting ducts. Thus, they indicate conditions exclusively within the kidneys and, for this reason, are of great diagnostic value. Except under the unusual conditions already mentioned, numerous casts are present only in renal disease.

Recent work suggests that the matrix of all casts is the high-molecular-weight Tamm-Horsfall mucoprotein.[28] Hyaline casts consist of this mucoprotein and appear as clear cylinders which are slightly refractile (Figures 20 and 20a). They dissolve readily in alkaline urine. Cellular elements may be incorporated into hyaline casts at the time of their formation. In this way, various types of casts are formed, depending on the cell type present. They may be red cells, white cells, epithelial cells, or combinations of all (Figures 21-23b). As the epithelial cells degenerate, casts become coarsely granular (Figures 24 and 24a), finely granular, and, finally, waxy in appearance (Figures 25 and 25a).

Broad casts come from collecting tubules (Figure 26). In large numbers they indicate the end-stage kidney.

White Cells and White-Cell Casts—The presence of an excess of white cells, singly or in clumps, in the urine indicates inflammation. The cause of the inflammation may be an infectious or noninfectious disease and may be located anywhere in the urinary system. White-cell casts (Figure 22) also indicate inflammation of unspecified origin but clearly pinpoint the kidneys as the disease site.

Although pyuria is a frequent finding in acute and chronic urinary tract infections and

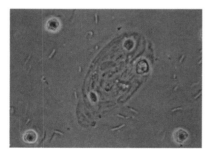

Figure 20. Hyaline cast, with RBC, WBC, and bacteria (phase-contrast microscope, 400×).

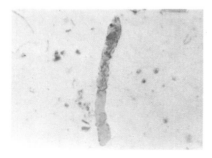

Figure 20a. Hyaline cast, Sternheimer–Malbin stain (standard light microscope, 400×).

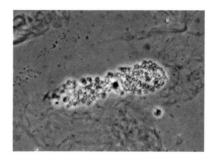

Figure 21. Red-cell cast (phase-contrast microscope, 400×).

is of great help in diagnosis, it is not a sufficient criterion of infection. Pyuria is the result of inflammation caused by a wide variety of noxious agents, including pathogenic bacteria. For example, it occurs in lupus nephritis as well as in radiation damage of the kidneys. In patients with acute appendicitis or with some pelvic inflammatory disease, the ureters may be affected by the inflammation outside the urinary tract. As a result, leukocytes may be present in a urine which is sterile. Also, white cells and white-cell clumps in the urine may be contaminants which have originated in the vagina or the prostate gland.

Following successful antimicrobial therapy, white blood cells and white-blood-cell casts may persist in the urine for many days, even though infection no longer exists in any part of the urinary system. However, persistent pyuria in a sterile urine should alert the physician to evaluate other causes of inflammation which are known to involve the kidneys and genito-urinary tract. Among these are anaerobic infections, tuberculosis, lupus nephritis and other forms of collagen disease, and renal tumor.

In patients having urine of relatively low specific gravity (e.g., 1.015) with little or no proteinuria and a scanty sediment, the physician should suspect chronic renal medullary

involvement and, particularly, chronic pyelonephritis. These patients may have a normal

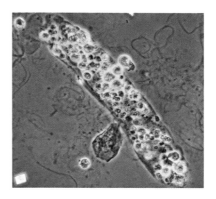

Figure 23. Mixed cellular cast with WBC and RBC and, to the left, a large epithelial cell (phase-contrast microscope, 400×).

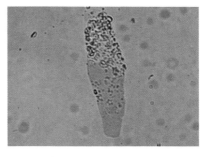

Figure 23a. Cellular cast, Sternheimer–Malbin stain (standard light microscope, 400×).

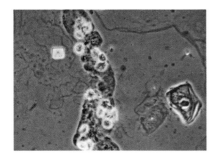

Figure 22. Finely granular white-cell cast, vaginal epithelium cell at right, and calcium oxalate crystal on left (phase-contrast microscope, 400×).

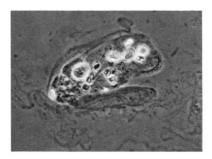

Figure 23b. Mixed cellular cast containing WBC, RBC, and an epithelial cell (phase-contrast microscope, 400×).

intravenous pyelogram. It may be necessary to examine the sediment from twenty or more urine specimens before white-cell casts are found to confirm the presence of inflammation of the kidneys.

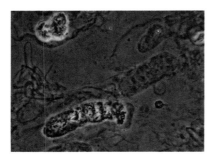

Figure 24. Granular cast (phase-contrast microscope, 400×).

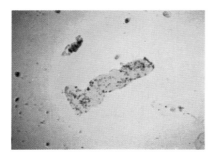

Figure 24a. Granular cast, Sternheimer–Malbin stain (standard light microscope, 400×).

Red Blood Cells and Red-Cell Casts—

Hematuria is not a hallmark of infection but nearly always accompanies the inflammatory process to a greater or lesser degree. Red blood cells may come from anywhere in the genito-urinary tract. They are lysed in dilute urine. Red-cell casts (Figure 21) originate in the kidney and usually indicate serious non-infective renal disease, such as glomerulo-nephritis, subacute bacterial endocarditis, and lupus nephritis or other collagen diseases.

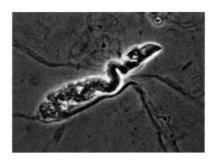

Figure 25. Half waxy and half granular cast (phase-contrast microscope, 400×).

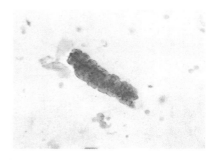

Figure 25a. Broad waxy cast, Sternheimer–Malbin stain (standard light microscope, 400×).

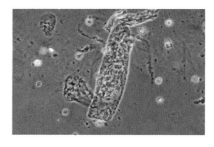

Figure 26. Broad granular cast (phase-contrast microscope, 400×).

Fats—

Oval fat bodies are remains of degenerated fat-filled tubular cells (Figure 27). They and fatty casts have no connection with infections of the kidneys or urinary tract but are found in the urine of patients with diabetic or other nephropathies. The predominant lipid in these structures is cholesterol ester (Figure 27a).

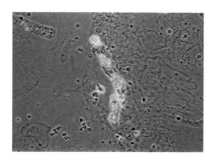

Figure 27. Oval fat bodies (phase-contrast micro-scope, 400✕).

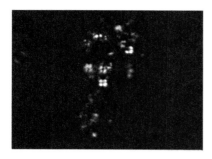

Figure 27a. When seen through a polarizing lens, the oval fat bodies appear as Maltese crosses, indicating cholesterol esters.

Crystalluria—In some metabolic diseases and in drug intoxications, characteristic crystals may appear in the urine. These are crystals of sulfonamides, cystine, leucine, tyrosine, and other amino acids. Crystals of urates are not specifically related to urinary tract infection and have little clinical significance.

RADIOLOGIC EXAMINATIONS

When continuous or recurrent significant bacteriuria is present or when renal infection is suspected for any reason, a complete radiologic evaluation of the urinary system is imperative. Several types of radiologic procedure are available.[29,30] Since each is intended to supply specific information, the choice of procedure to be used depends on the patient's suspected disorder. However, in almost all cases, the examination is begun with plain radiography and intravenous pyelography.

Plain Radiography of Abdomen and Pelvis—The flat plate, or "scout" film, provides evidence of calcification within the kidneys due, for example, to tuberculous lesions or nephrocalcinosis. It reveals also any radiopaque objects, such as calculi and other foreign bodies, in the kidneys or elsewhere in the urinary tract (Figure 28). However, oblique views usually are required for clear differentiation of calculi in the kidneys or pelves from gallstones and calcified mesenteric glands. The scout film should be examined for evidence of other diseases of the kidneys and genito-urinary tract, such as tumors, cysts, or hydronephrosis. Evidence of bone lesions, tumors in the pelvic or retroperitoneal space, or abdominal lesions that displace or impinge on the genito-urinary tract may be seen in the flat plate. These x-ray films should always precede the intravenous pyelograms.

Intravenous Pyelography—When a contrast medium is injected intravenously, it is excreted by the kidney in sufficient concentration to make the urine radiopaque. Therefore, with radiopaque urine in the kidneys, renal pelves, ureters, and bladder, these structures are visible in the roentgenogram.

The standard intravenous pyelogram (IVP) or excretory urogram serves many purposes (Figure 29). It can establish the presence and position of the kidneys and evaluate their size and shape. It is also useful in demonstrating congenital or acquired abnormalities in any portion of the urinary system and in the structures which impinge on it (Figure 30).

Intravenous pyelography gives gross information on the functional state of the kidneys

Figure 28. Plain AP film of abdomen showing nephrolithiasis—staghorn calculi of left renal pelvis and multiple calculi of right collecting system.

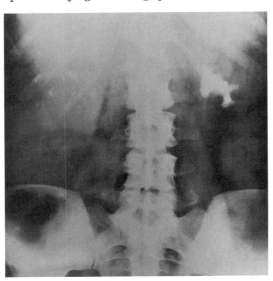
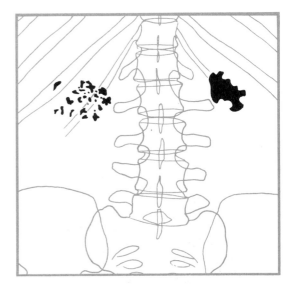

Figure 29. IVP of twenty-four-year-old female, showing normal structures.

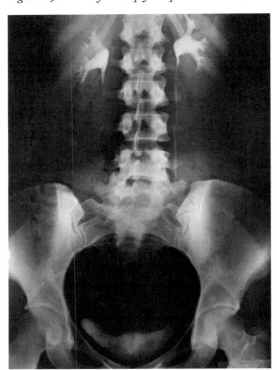
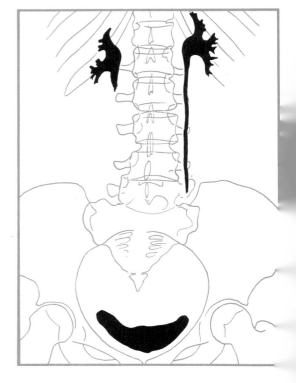

Figure 30. IVP showing a normal collecting system on the left. There is a double collecting system on the right which clears less contrast media; this indicates the presence of a vascular lesion.

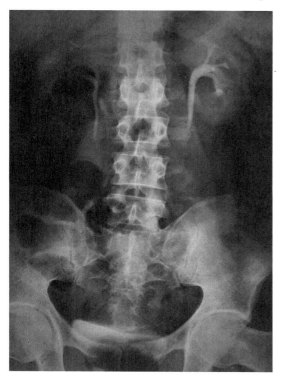
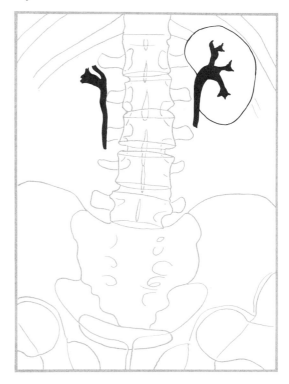

and other portions of the urinary system. For example, in acute pyelonephritis, the kidneys are swollen and are measurably larger in films exposed during the infection than in those taken six weeks after treatment. The decrease in size may be two or more centimeters, and it clearly indicates the disappearance of inflammatory exudate and edema.

In infants and children, intravenous pyelography is usually postponed until the infection has been brought under control. However, if dribbling, an enlarged bladder, or an abdominal mass is present (suggesting that the urinary tract infection is secondary to obstructive uropathy), the intravenous pyelogram should not be delayed. Intravenous

pyelography is indicated in newborn infants with clinical evidence of gross congenital abnormalities of the urinary tract, such as epispadias or hypospadias.

In chronic pyelonephritis, one or both of the kidneys may be small. Scars may be evident. Infiltration of fatty tissue may occur and will appear on the film as coarse dark bands in the medulla and juxtamedullary cortex. Distortion of the renal pelvis with "clubbing" is a common finding (Figure 31) but is not pathognomonic for pyelonephritis, as has been stated. It may be seen with various forms of chronic renal involvement, such as renal artery stenosis and renal hypoplasia, in which evidence of infection is lacking.

Figure 31. IVP showing clubbing of calyces without shrinkage, which suggests pyelonephritis.

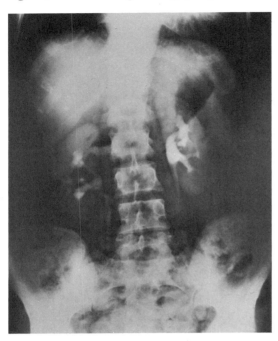 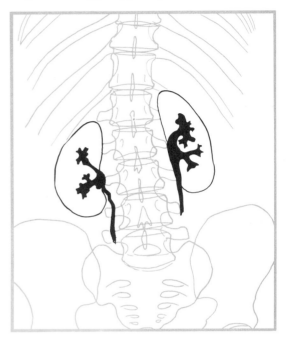

Figure 32. Rapid-sequence urography one minute after injection of dye. Delayed nephrogram on right side indicates arterial vascular disease.

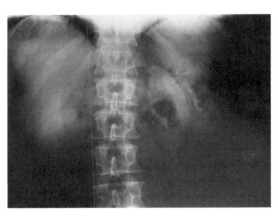 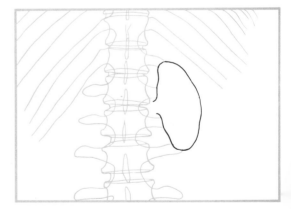

Timed Excretory Urography—By use of this procedure, the effect of different disease states on the kidney's ability to concentrate and excrete dye is measured. Briefly, x-ray films are exposed at specified intervals (1, 3, 4, 5, and 10 minutes) after intravenous injection of a radiopaque dye. In this way, the rate of dye concentration by the kidneys (Figures 32 and 33) and the time of its appearance in the pelves and ureters are determined

(Figures 33–33e). Since it is possible to obtain such data for each kidney separately, comparisons between the two kidneys may be made. Timed excretory urography is particularly useful whenever one kidney is found to be smaller than the other. This discrepancy in size may be due to hyperplasia, unilateral renal artery disease, or unilateral chronic infection and is noted in certain rare conditions, such as medullary sponge kidney.

Timed excretory urography is a useful screening procedure in detecting renal artery stenosis in hypertensive patients. Since renal artery stenosis results in increased water reabsorption, volume is reduced, which causes dye to be concentrated in the affected kidney but not in the other.

Similar concentration of dye does not take place with "pure" unilateral chronic pyelonephritis. The increased dye concentration is readily evident on the x-ray film in the unusually intense opacity or "whiteness" of the pelvis and ureter.

Angionephrotomography

Angionephrotomography—This procedure is done with or without a radiopaque dye. Its purpose is to show the kidneys in "cross section" and to reveal any cysts or other abnormalities which may be present. Tomography also gives a useful first approximation of kidney size, if such information has not already been obtained from the intravenous pyelogram. However, for this purpose, massive-dose intravenous pyelography is usually the preferred technic.

Massive-Dose Intravenous Pyelography

Massive-Dose Intravenous Pyelography—In chronic renal failure, when glomerular and tubular functions are severely depressed, the kidneys cannot concentrate dye. Accordingly, it may be necessary to use five or six times the standard dose of dye in a glucose solution and infuse it intravenously over a period of thirty to sixty minutes to visualize the kidneys, pelves, and ureters.

The infusion technic is also very useful for filling pelves and ureters in patients with little or no loss of renal function, because it may show details in these structures well enough to make retrograde cystographic examination unnecessary. Its use should be considered whenever possible to replace the retrograde procedure.

Selective Renal Angiography

Selective Renal Angiography—Renal arteriograms are of prime importance in the diagnosis of renal tumors and constitute a very necessary part of the study of patients with hypertension who are suspected of having some form of renal artery stenosis.

Small kidneys may result from congenital hypoplasia or from contraction due to infection or to renal artery stenosis. The resulting distortion of the pelves, as revealed by intravenous pyelography, may appear the same, regardless of etiology. To determine the origin of the small kidney, use is made of selective renal angiography.[31] In this procedure, special instruments and catheters are used to inject a radiopaque dye into each renal artery.

In the hypoplastic kidney, the diameter of the opening of the renal artery where it leaves the abdominal aorta is small. The renal artery is also small and smooth, with parallel walls throughout its entire length. In essence, a hypoplastic arterial system supplies a hypoplastic kidney.

The artery to a kidney contracted because of infection is also contracted. However, the original diameter is retained at its aortic origin, but this diminishes rapidly toward the kidney. Therefore, the artery is said to resemble a cone, and "coning down" is considered to be of diagnostic significance.

Figure 33. Rapid-sequence urography. Plain film showing kidneys of normal size without calculi.

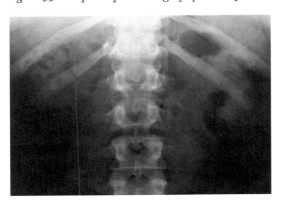 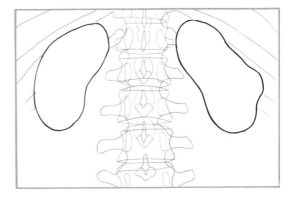

Figure 33a. One minute after injection of radiopaque dye. Normal nephrogram.

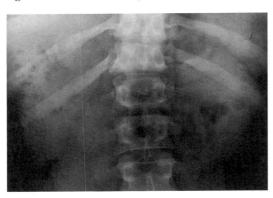 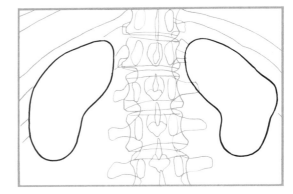

Figure 33b. Three minutes after injection. Symmetrical homogenous nephrogram with kidneys of equal size.

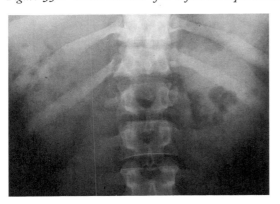 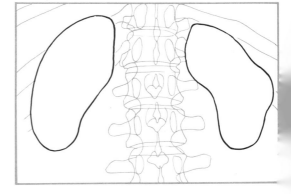

Figure 33c. Four minutes after injection, contrast is seen in both kidneys.

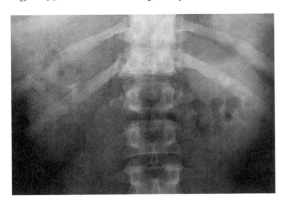 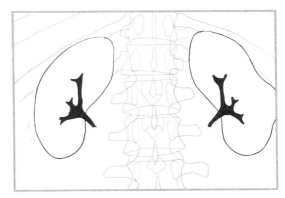

Figure 33d. Five minutes after injection, symmetrical calyceal system; i.e., each kidney is clearing the same amount of dye.

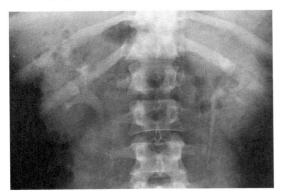 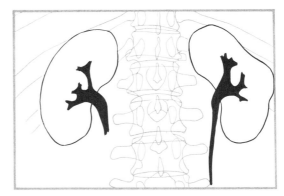

Figure 33e. Ten minutes after injection, the collecting systems are normal.

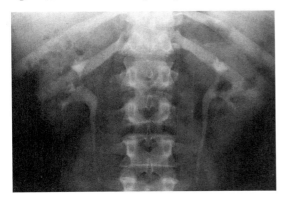 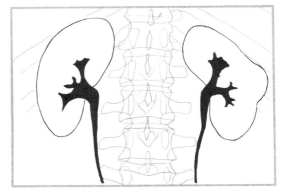

When the kidney is small because of renal artery lesion, the stenosis is evident, as sometimes is the poststenotic dilatation of the involved renal artery (Figure 34).

Retrograde Radiography—In retrograde radiography, a radiopaque dye is injected into the renal pelvis. This is done through a ureteral catheter which has been positioned in the renal pelvis or as high up the ureter as possible. The procedure is valuable for locating the site of an obstruction and indicating the details of any abnormalities in the upper portions of the ureters and the pelves. Clubbing, stone, fibrosis, papilloma, papillary necrosis, ureteral-pelvic junction anomalies, tuberculosis, and the so-called medullary sponge kidneys are revealed by the retrograde technic (Figure 35).

The retrograde examination can be combined with cystoscopy, which is a most important diagnostic function of the urologic surgeon. If necessary, urine can be collected from each ureter separately for culture and urinalysis. By use of specially designed ureteral catheters, urine samples can be obtained simultaneously at specified intervals from the left and right kidneys. Data on the concentration, rate of excretion, and clearances of sodium, creatinine, and aminohippuric acid can be obtained by appropriate analyses of these samples.

Cystourethrography—Abnormalities in the lower urinary tract, particularly bladder-neck obstructions and reflux, are detected on the voiding cystourethrogram. Dye is injected into the bladder via a urethral catheter or percutaneous needle, and the urinary tract is examined with multiple views. The posterior urethra, bladder neck, bladder, vesicoureteral junction, and the ureters may be examined before, during, and after voiding. Cinematography, television, and kinescopes, with or

Figure 34. Selective injection of the left renal artery, showing an area of stenosis with poststenotic dilatation.

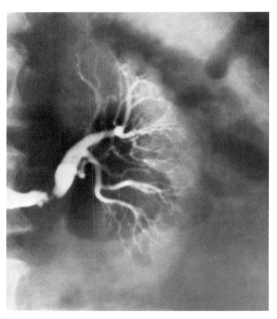
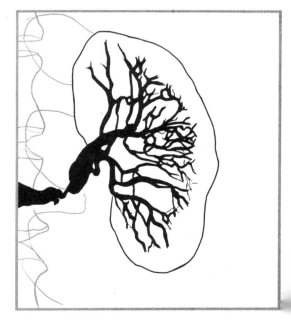

Figure 35. Retrograde pyelogram showing tuberculosis in right kidney.

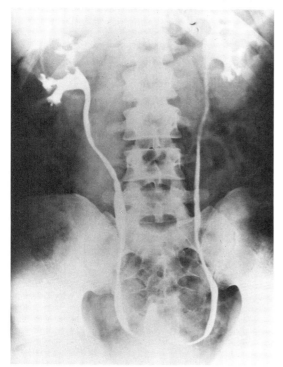
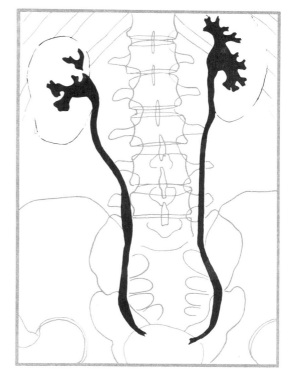

without magnification, are useful for this purpose (Figures 36-39).

In some centers, cystourethrography is done routinely on all women with an initial attack of proved urinary tract infection, because it provides information on the nature of the vesicoureteral reflux, if present, and reveals any posterior urethral obstruction. In most cases, this examination should be done after the urinary tract infection has been brought under control. If the examination is made soon after the infection is controlled, however, abnormal results may be seen, because an infection nearly always induces transient bilateral vesicoureteral reflux. At least two weeks should elapse after the infection is cured before voiding cystourethrography is done. Should the reflux persist for more than three months after successful therapy,

further urologic study should be undertaken.

RENAL BIOPSY

Percutaneous needle biopsy is an uncertain diagnostic procedure in pyelonephritis.[32,33] Because of the uneven involvement of the kidney and the small size of the biopsy sample —about 25 glomeruli from approximately one million—an affected area may be missed and only normal tissue obtained. Furthermore, even if the renal disease is extensive, microscopic examination alone may not distinguish changes due to infection from those of other etiology. In the opinion of some authorities, renal biopsy is contraindicated in kidney infections and, in general, should not be undertaken until all other methods have failed to yield a diagnosis.

Figure 36. Normal cystogram in a twenty-four-year-old female.

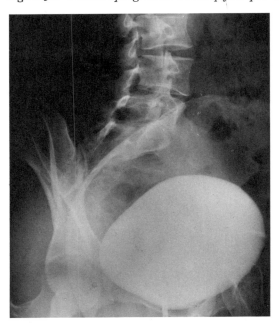 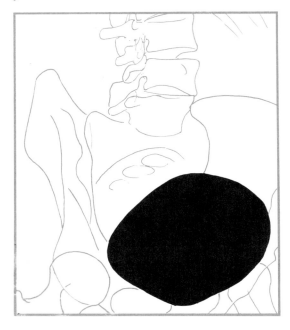

Figure 37. Cystogram showing bilateral vesicoureteral reflux which is more marked on the right.

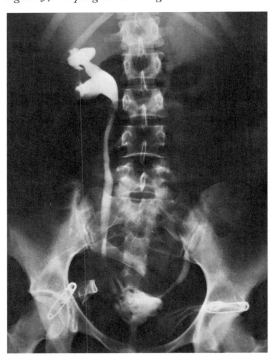 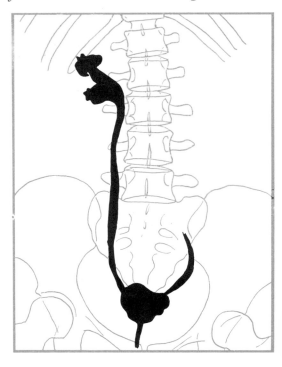

Figure 38. Cystogram showing bilateral ureteral reflux in a five-year-old female.

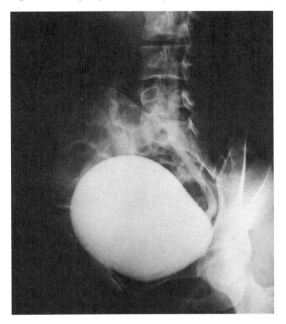 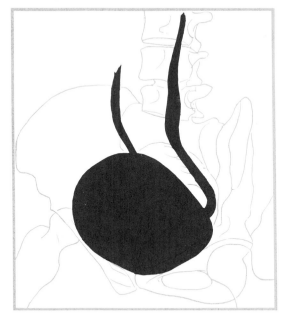

Figure 39. Cystogram showing trabeculation of bladder dome.

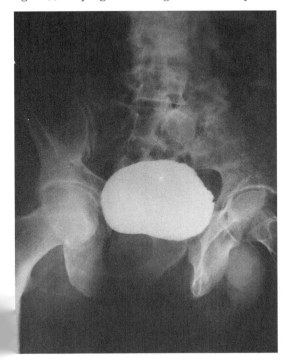 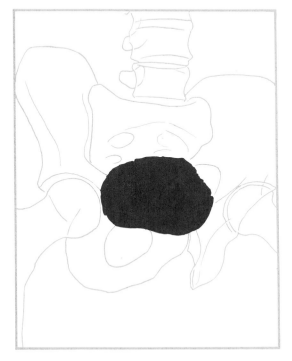

BOX 2

MORPHOLOGIC CRITERIA OF PYELONEPHRITIS

Pyelonephritis may affect one or both kidneys. When only one kidney is involved, its weight may be reduced to 20 or 30 Gm. If involvement of both kidneys occurs, often one kidney is affected more than the other.

Examination of the whole kidney reveals numerous coarse depressions—i.e., scars—on the subcapsular surface (a). The intervening areas are smooth, but they may be finely granular when intrarenal artery disease is present.

A cut section of the kidney shows that the surface depressions correspond to areas where the parenchyma is thin and scarred (b). There, the papillae are blunted and retracted; the calyces are dilated and club-shaped. Numerous calyces may be affected, although changes are confined to a single calyceal system in some cases. Parenchymal scars and dilated calyces are characteristic of pyelonephritis. A thorough inspection of the pelvicalyceal system is therefore essential, and its relation to parenchymal scars should be noted.

Microscopic examination of tissue sections from scarred areas reveals a profoundly altered parenchyma. Glomeruli may be considerably reduced in size or completely obliterated by an accumulation of collagen-like material in Bowman's capsule (c); or, the glomeruli may become structureless—i.e., undergo hyalinization—without change in Bowman's capsule. In less severely affected portions, periglomerular fibrosis occurs but is sparing of glomeruli (d); that is, the collagen-like material is seen deposited in rings surrounding Bowman's capsule.

Tubules (for the most part, these are collecting ducts) in the scarred areas are dilated and, character-istically, consist of atrophied epithelium in which cells are noticeably flattened. The lumen contains homogenous eosinophilic casts, often called "colloid casts." The presence of such tubules and the exclusion of other normal parenchymal structures simulate thyroid tissue in appearance; accordingly, these changes are described as "thyroidization" (e). In less affected portions, tubules may contain polymorphonuclear leukocytes.

The interstitium is usually fibrotic, with lymphocytes, plasma cells, and, in some cases, eosinophils.

Cells characteristic of chronic inflammation are common in calyceal and pelvic epithelium, which may be thickened. Lymphoid follicles with well-developed germinal centers may also be present.

Alterations in arteries are varied. In some, there may be virtually none; in others, there may be a marked degree of fibrous intimal thickening.

Areas of tissue with the alterations in morphology described above characteristically occur in patches separated by parenchyma which is normal in appearance. This is seen in f, where the transition from old infected area (right) to normal area (left) is abrupt.

(Illustrations a, b, e, and f from Heptinstall, R. H.: Pathology of the Kidney. Boston: Little, Brown & Company, 1966. Courtesy of the author and publisher.)

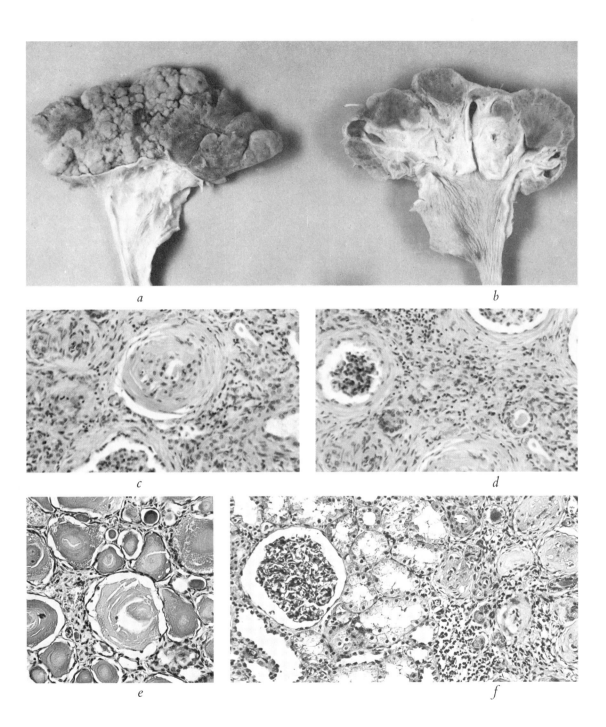

a

b

c

d

e

f

BIBLIOGRAPHY

1. Kunin, C. M., Petersdorf, R. G., Kimmelstiel, P., and Relman, A. S.: Asymptomatic Bacteriuria: Significance and Management, in Controversy in Internal Medicine (edited by F. J. Ingelfinger, A. S. Relman, and M. Finland), p. 289. Philadelphia: W. B. Saunders Company, 1966.

2. Kass, E. H.: Asymptomatic Infections of the Urinary Tract, Tr. A. Am. Physicians, 69:56, 1956.

3. Kunin, C. M., Zacha, E., and Paquin, A. J., Jr.: Urinary Tract Infections in School Children. I. Prevalence of Bacteriuria and Associated Urologic Findings, New England J. Med., 266:1287, 1962.

4. Kaitz, A. L., and Williams, E. J.: Bacteriuria and Urinary Tract Infections in Hospitalized Patients, New England J. Med., 262:425, 1960.

5. Kass, E. H.: Personal communication.

6. Stamey, T. A., Govan, D. E., and Palmer, J. M.: The Localization and Treatment of Urinary Tract Infections: The Role of Bactericidal Urine Levels as Opposed to Serum Levels, Medicine, 44:1, 1965.

7. Saccharow, L., and Pryles, C. V.: Further Experience with the Use of Percutaneous Suprapubic Aspiration of the Urinary Bladder; Bacteriologic Studies in 654 Infants and Children, Pediatrics, 43:1018, 1969.

8. Kark, R. M.: Personal communication.

9. Kunin, C. M.: The Quantitative Significance of Bacteria Visualized in the Unstained Urinary Sediment, New England J. Med., 265:589, 1961.

10. Brody, L., Webster, M. C., and Kark, R. M.: Identification of Elements of Urinary Sediment with Phase-Contrast Microscopy, J.A.M.A., 206:1777, 1968.

11. Cohen, S. N., and Kass, E. H.: A Simple Method for Quantitative Urine Culture, New England J. Med., 277:176, 1967.

12. Kass, E. H.: Bacteriuria and the Diagnosis of Infections of the Urinary Tract, Arch. Int. Med., 100:709, 1957.

13. Kass, E. H.: Bacteriuria and the Pathogenesis of Pyelonephritis, Lab. Invest., 9:110, 1960.

14. Neter, E.: Evaluation of the Tetrazolium Test for the Diagnosis of Significant Bacteriuria, J.A.M.A., 192:769, 1965.

15. Finnerty, F. A., Jr., and Johnson, A. C.: A Simplified Accurate Method for Detecting Bacteriuria, Am. J. Obst. & Gynec., 101:238, 1968.

16. Dubach, U. C.: Enzymes in Kidney and Urine. Baltimore: The Williams & Wilkins Company, 1968.

17. Kark, R. M., Lawrence, J. R., Pollak, V. E., Pirani, C. L., Muehrcke, R. C., and Silva, H.: A Primer of Urinalysis, Ed. 2. New York: Hoeber Medical Division, Harper & Row, Publishers, 1963.

18. Wolf, A. V., and Pillay, V. K. G.: Renal Concentration Tests: Osmotic Pressure, Specific Gravity, Refraction, and Electrical Conductivity Compared, Am. J. Med., 46:837, 1969.

19. Kaitz, A. L.: Urinary Concentrating Ability in Pregnant Women with Asymptomatic Bacteriuria, J. Clin. Invest., 40:1331, 1961.

20. Gellman, D. D., Pirani, C. L., Soothill, J. F., Muehrcke, R. C., and Kark, R. M.: Diabetic Nephropathy: A Clinical and Pathologic Study Based on Renal Biopsies, Medicine, 38:321, 1959.

21. Thomsen, A. C.: The Kidney in Diabetes Mellitus. Copenhagen: Ejnar Munksgaards Forlag, 1965.

22. Rowe, D. S., and Soothill, J. F.: Serum Proteins in Normal Urine, Clin. Sc., 21:75, 1961.

23. Rowe, D. S., and Soothill, J. F.: The Proteins of Postural and Exercise Proteinuria, Clin. Sc., 21:87, 1961.

24. Cameron, J. S., and Blandford, G.: The Simple Assessment of Selectivity in Heavy Proteinuria, Lancet, 2:242, 1966.

25. Kark, R. M.: Personal communication.

26. Kark, R. M.: Personal communication.

27. Prescott, L. F., and Brodie, D. E.: A Simple Differential Stain for Urinary Sediment, Lancet, 2:940, 1964.

28. McQueen, E. G., and Sidney, M. B.: Composition of Urinary Casts, Lancet, 1:397, 1966.

29. Ney, A., and Friedenberg, R. N.: Radiographic Atlas of the Genito-Urinary System. Philadelphia: J. B. Lippincott Company, 1966.

30. Alken, C. E., Dix, V. W., Goodwin, W. E., and Wildbolz, E.: Encyclopedia of Urology, V. Part 1. Diagnostic Radiology. Berlin: Springer-Verlag, 1962.

31. Kincaid, O. W., and Davis, G. D.: Renal Angiography. Chicago: Year Book Medical Publishers, Inc., 1966.

32. Brun, C., Raaschone, F., and Eriksen, K. R.: Simultaneous Bacteriologic Studies of Renal Biopsies and Urine, in Progress in Pyelonephritis (edited by E. H. Kass), p. 461. Philadelphia: F. A. Davis Company, 1965.

33. Pawlowski, J. M., Bloxdorf, J. W., and Kimmelstiel, P.: Chronic Pyelonephritis; A Morphologic and Bacteriologic Study, New England J. Med., 268:965, 1963.

GENERAL REFERENCES

Becker, E. L. (Editor): Structural Basis of Renal Disease. New York: Hoeber Medical Division, Harper & Row, Publishers, 1968.

Black, M. M., and Wagner, B. M.: Dynamic Pathology; Structural and Functional Mechanisms of Disease. St. Louis: C. V. Mosby Company, 1964.

Heptinstall, R. H.: Pathology of the Kidney. Boston: Little, Brown & Company, 1966.

Ingelfinger, F. J., Relman, A. S., and Finland, M. (Editors): Controversy in Internal Medicine. Philadelphia: W. B. Saunders Company, 1966.

Moyer, J. H., and Swartz, C. D. (Guest Editors): Treatment of Pyelonephritis, Mod. Treat., 7:256 (March), 1970.

Strauss, M. B., and Welt, L. G. (Editors): Diseases of the Kidney. Boston: Little, Brown & Company, 1963.

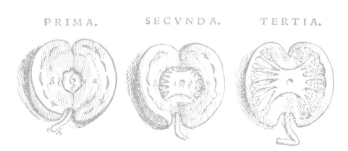

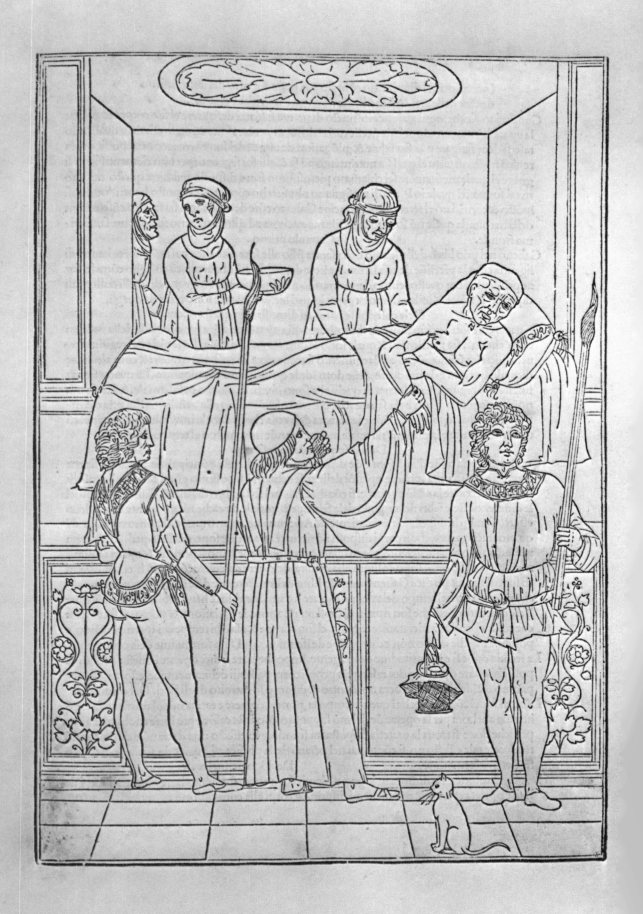

4
The Patient

THE SYMPTOMATIC PATIENT

Some patients with kidney or urinary tract infection seek medical help because they do not feel well. Their complaints cover a broad range of symptoms and account for the diversity of physicians likely to be consulted.

Significance of Signs and Symptoms—The symptomatic patient may be the individual who feels tired all the time or who says he has the "flu," the child who begins wetting after having been toilet-trained, or the woman with low-back pain. Even after detailed questioning, such patients may deny any symptoms referable to the urinary tract, and physical examination may not reveal any specific abnormalities.

physician examining his patient while protecting himself from infection by a sponge impregnated with aromatic ces held to his nose and mouth. The attendant on the right holds a urine carrier.

Joannes de: Fasciculus medicinae. Venice, 1493. (Courtesy of the Lilly Library, Indiana University, Bloomington, Indiana)

Table 3 *SIGNS AND SYMPTOMS OFTEN ACCOMPANYING BACTERIURIA*

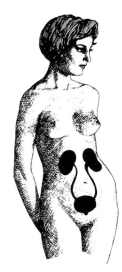

In the
Acutely Ill Patient—

Hematuria
Fever, chills
Dysuria, urgency, frequency
Back pain
Abdominal pain

In the
Chronically Ill Patient—

Low-back pain
Nocturia
Easy fatigability
Anorexia, weight loss
Growth disturbances (in children)

In other instances, the diagnosis will be obvious. The patient complains of pain on urination. The pain is sometimes mild, sometimes excruciatingly severe. This may be accompanied by gross hematuria, and, usually, frequency of urination and nocturia are present. Back pain may be mild and nonspecific, or it may be severe. The pain may be located anteriorly for the most part and be difficult to distinguish from such abdominal conditions as acute cholecystitis or acute appendicitis. The temperature varies widely; it may be normal or reach 105°F. Shaking chills may also occur. Some subjects will have symptoms of renal insufficiency, with nausea, vomiting, itching of the skin, weight loss, weakness, edema, and shortness of breath (Table 3).

THE ASYMPTOMATIC PATIENT

Upon routine urinalysis, patients with other illnesses or those undergoing health checkups and examinations or participating in surveys frequently are found to have a urinary tract infection. Still another group will be inves-

tigated because of the finding of hypertension or its complications. Finally, it is now customary also to culture the urine of pregnant women, and positive results can be anticipated in about 3 to 8 percent of cultures. A summary appears in Table 4.

Significance of Signs and Symptoms—Although the preceding patients are generally spoken of as "asymptomatic," a surprising number of them admit upon questioning to

Table 4

DISCOVERY OF BACTERIURIA
IN THE ASYMPTOMATIC
PATIENT MAY OCCUR
BECAUSE OF ROUTINE
URINALYSIS IN:

Health checkup
Diagnosis of other illness
Hypertension and complications
Pregnancy
Population surveys
Insurance or employment examinations

episodes of symptoms separated by asymptomatic intervals. An occasional individual will be unaware of not feeling well until he experiences the well-being which often follows successful treatment.

Generally, when the physician considers the possibility of urinary tract infection, the symptoms are not sufficient to establish the diagnosis because they are nonspecific and could easily be due to some other cause. This is particularly true in infants and young children in whom gastro-intestinal symptoms may predominate and in whom, on occasion, the only sign of infection may be failure to thrive.

Whether or not to attribute a particular set of signs or symptoms to urinary infections after bacteriuria is established is often a difficult decision. For example, patients with chronic bacteriuria may also develop acute appendicitis, gall-bladder disease, or acute glomerulonephritis. Care must be taken not to attribute too much to the presence of urinary tract infection. This is a particular problem in patients with preexisting renal disease when the histological findings are consistent with those of chronic pyelonephritis but may as well be those of diabetic nephropathy, arteriolosclerosis, nephrocalcinosis, or obstructive uropathy (Figure 40). The mere association of urinary tract infection and a disease of the kidney does not by any means establish a causal relationship.

DIAGNOSIS AND MANAGEMENT

Physical Examination—No abnormalities may be found upon physical examination. On the other hand, tenderness over the bladder, ureters, or kidneys (anteriorly and posteriorly) may be severe. Kidney tenderness in some instances may be so "exquisite" as to satisfy the criteria for peritonitis.

Figure 40. Sites and incidence of obstruction in the urinary tract.

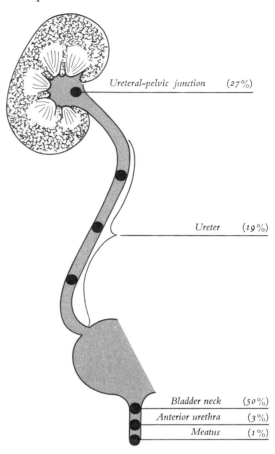

Ureteral-pelvic junction   (27%)

Ureter   (19%)

Bladder neck   (50%)
Anterior urethra   (3%)
Meatus   (1%)

Bacteriuria—Detailed consideration of bacteriologic and other laboratory procedures useful in diagnosis and interpretation of findings is included elsewhere (see Chapter 3). It is important to emphasize at this point, however, that the *presence or absence of bacteriuria must be determined before a decision is made regarding therapy and subsequent management of the patient.* Only in the occasional acutely ill patient should it be necessary to start antibiotic therapy before the presence of bacteria in the urine is established. Table 5 lists the

Table 5

SPECIFIC CIRCUMSTANCES
REQUIRING SEARCH FOR
BACTERIURIA

Table 5

SPECIFIC CIRCUMSTANCES REQUIRING SEARCH FOR BACTERIURIA

Pregnancy, especially with history of toxemia
Diabetes mellitus
Hypertension
Anemia
Age of sixty and over
Hematuria, proteinuria
Excessive use of phenacetin
Prior genito-urinary abnormality or instrumentation
Deafness or renal disease in family

specific circumstances requiring that a search for bacteriuria be made.

Antimicrobial Therapy—One of the commonest errors made in the management of patients suspected of having urinary infections is institution of expensive and sometimes dangerous therapy before the diagnosis has been properly established. The procedure chosen depends largely on the specific circumstances encountered. If the patient has few or no symptoms, it is best to await the results of urine culture and confirm them before starting therapy. For example, dysuria, if present, may perhaps be caused by a low urinary pH and can usually be alleviated by 1/2 teaspoonful of sodium bicarbonate in a glass of water taken as needed for a day or two until administration of specific antibiotics can begin.

On the other hand, if the patient is severely ill (high fever or signs of peritonitis), admission to a hospital may be mandatory, with antibiotic therapy given at once. Of course, symptoms may warrant starting antibiotic therapy without hospital admission.

There is no perfect antimicrobial agent for kidney and urinary tract infections. The clinician's goal is to use the agent that will be most effective against the offending microorganism at the site of infection. Drugs differ so greatly in toxicity that possible side-effects which may complicate therapy must be weighed against the severity of illness. Thus, the patient with dysuria but without systemic symptoms would not need the same type of antimicrobial agent as the patient with an indwelling catheter who is known to be infected with *Pseudomonas* and who suddenly develops chills, fever, and hypertension. A relatively nontoxic oral drug would be indicated in the former case whereas, in the latter, parenteral treatment with drugs (indicated by the previously established in-vitro sensitivity of the organism) would be mandatory. (Further discussion of antimicrobial therapy occurs in Chapter 5.)

Remission of Signs and Symptoms—It is well known that urinary and kidney infections are often self-limited; the signs and symptoms will normally subside in three to four days—with or without therapy. Therefore, *prompt remission of symptoms per se cannot be taken as an indication of successful eradication of bacteriuria.* Conversely, in some patients with uncomplicated, nonobstructive acute pyelonephritis, fever and kidney tenderness may persist for seven to ten days despite effective antimicrobial therapy. In general, however, when fever and kidney pain and tenderness do not subside within three or four days, it is important to look for some underlying lesion of the genito-urinary system by means of intravenous pyelography.

Laboratory Findings—If effective and appropriate antimicrobial agents are being used, the urine should become sterile within two to three days, but pyuria and hematuria may continue for considerably longer periods of time (see Urine Culture during Therapy, page 78). In particular, patients with papillary necrosis or renal stones may have pyuria for weeks after the urine has become sterilized. However, one must always be alert to the possibility that persistent pyuria indicates inadequate antibiotic therapy or, perhaps, underlying genito-urinary tuberculosis.

Although gross hematuria is common at the time of acute infection, red cells should disappear when the urine becomes sterile. The persistence of hematuria in a patient who is asymptomatic, with or without infection, is strongly suggestive that some other lesion is present in the genito-urinary system (such as stone, glomerulonephritis, or tumor).

THE CLINICAL COURSE OF THE DISEASE

Cure and Relapse—About 50 percent of patients treated for one to two weeks with effective antimicrobial agents will have sterile urine cultures one to two years later.[1,2] In a like period, the remainder will suffer a relapse with the same organism or, more commonly, will be reinfected with a different one. Since these relapses or reinfections are usually asymptomatic for variable intervals before symptoms develop, it is necessary to follow up on patients with urine cultures for prolonged periods after treatment is completed. For example, some physicians obtain urine cultures after three and six weeks and then at three, six, and twelve months.

Relapse in Men and Women—If a female patient has had two or three episodes of urinary infection, she should be investigated more thoroughly; e.g., blood urea nitrogen should be determined, and an intravenous pyelogram should be done. *In men, because of the relative rarity of genito-urinary infections, it is advisable to carry out intravenous pyelography after the first infection.*

In the opinion of many physicians, the voiding cystourethrogram should be done on any patient with recurrent infection, even though the intravenous pyelogram is normal. It must be noted, however, that there is a great deal of uncertainty as to the significance of such abnormalities as meatal stenosis, urethral stenosis, megalocystis, and bladder-neck obstruction and that repair of these ill-defined conditions favorably influences the clinical course of the infection.[3]

Sources of Bacteriuria—Some authorities consider the source of bacteriuria to be an important factor in the future course of an infection. For example, it is believed that a recurrent infection with the same organism is more likely to occur when the bacteriuria originates in the upper urinary tract, whereas reinfection with a new organism is the stronger possibility when the infection is confined to the bladder.[4]

Determining the site of infection is useful for investigative purposes, but it is not recommended for the routine management of patients.[4] The procedure involves ureteral catheterization and hence the risk of transporting bacteria from the bladder to the kidney. By this means, bladder bacteriuria on one day could easily become pyelonephritis on the next. In support of this is the observation that many women experience dysuria some days prior to the appearance of full-blown acute pyelonephritis. Catheterization may also be the means of spreading bacteria from other locations. In men, the prostate is a proved source of recurrent urinary infection

Figure 41. The risks of renal damage in urinary tract infections.

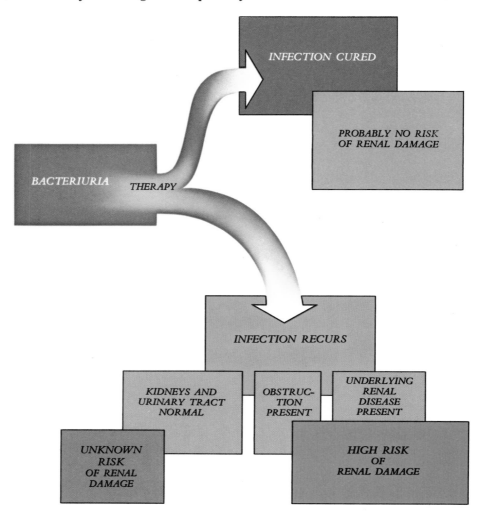

with the same organism.[5] The paraurethral glands in women may play a similar role, although this has not been verified.

Prognosis—The widespread appreciation of the value of quantitative urine culture is so recent that adequately documented follow-up studies on significant numbers of patients are scarce. It is known that the urine in a certain number of patients will become sterile with-

out antibiotic therapy.[1,2] In many others, however, recurrent or persistent infections will continue (Figure 41).

The long-term consequences of urinary infection in patients without underlying disorders are not certain, since relatively few have been studied and the period of follow-up has been short (Figure 41).

In some patients with persistent or recurrent urinary infections of ten or more years' duration, it may not be possible to detect, by x-ray, by signs of renal functional impairment, or by the development of hypertension, evidence of progressive kidney destruction. Furthermore, in almost all patients with evidence of renal impairment or hypertension, there has been some additional disorder or condition (by itself capable of producing renal damage) associated with the infection. Examples are obstruction, diabetes, hypertension, or analgesic ingestion (Figure 41).

Past studies of autopsy material were once considered convincing in suggesting that, in the absence of underlying disease, chronic renal insufficiency might result from silent urinary infections. Careful review of these data casts doubt on the conclusion that the renal disease was, in fact, due to infection.[6] Although the matter is not settled, a preliminary study of patients with documented renal infections does not lend support to this view.

Summary—Patients with urinary tract infections and pyelonephritis are likely to be seen by many kinds of physicians and to be detected under various circumstances. Some patients will have life-threatening infections; others will be unaware of any symptoms.

It is essential to establish the presence of bacteria in the urine before treatment is undertaken. *Disappearance of symptoms cannot be relied upon to indicate bacteriologic cure.* To be meaningful, follow-up must extend over long periods of time and must include frequent bacteriologic examinations of the urine.

There are many unresolved questions concerning the natural history and clinical course of these infections. It is apparent, however, that proper surveillance and careful follow-up will always be necessary.

BIBLIOGRAPHY

1. Freedman, L. R., Seki, M., and Phair, J. P.: The Natural History and Outcome of Antibiotic Treatment of Urinary Tract Infections in Women, Yale J. Biol. & Med., *37*:245, 1965.

2. Asscher, A. W., Sussman, M., Waters, W. E., Evans, J. A. S., Campbell, H., Evans, D. T., and Williams, J. E.: Asymptomatic Significant Bacteriuria in the Non-Pregnant Woman. II. Response to Treatment and Follow-up, Brit. M. J., *1*:804, 1969.

3. Glenn, J. F. (Editor): Workshop in Ureteral Reflux in Children. Washington: National Academy of Sciences/National Research Council, 1966.

4. Turck, M., Anderson, K. N., and Petersdorf, R. G.: Relapse and Reinfection in Chronic Bacteriuria, New England J. Med., *275*:70, 1966.

5. Meares, E. M., and Stamey, T. A.: Bacteriologic Localization Patterns in Bacterial Prostatitis and Urethritis, Invest. Urol., *5*:492, 1968.

6. Freedman, L. R.: Chronic Pyelonephritis at Autopsy, Ann. Int. Med., *66*:697, 1967.

GENERAL REFERENCES

Freedman, L. R.: Pyelonephritis and Urinary Tract Infection, in Diseases of the Kidney (edited by M. B. Strauss and L. G. Welt), p. 469. Boston: Little, Brown & Company, 1963.

Guze, L. B., and Beeson, P. B.: Observations on the Reliability and Safety of Bladder Catheterization for Bacteriologic Study of the Urine, New England J. Med., *255*:474, 1956.

Kunin, C. M., and McCormack, R. C.: Prevention of Catheter-Induced Urinary-Tract Infections by Sterile Closed Drainage, New England J. Med., *274*:1155, 1966.

Montgomerie, J. Z., Kalmanson, G. M., and Guze, L. B.: Renal Failure and Infection, Medicine, *47*:1, 1968.

Norden, C. W., and Kass, E. H.: Bacteriuria of Pregnancy—A Critical Appraisal, Ann. Rev. Med., *19*: 431, 1968.

Petersdorf, R. G.: Asymptomatic Bacteriuria: A Therapeutic Enigma, in Controversy in Internal Medicine (edited by F. J. Ingelfinger, A. S. Relman, and M. Finland), p. 302. Philadelphia: W. B. Saunders Company, 1966.

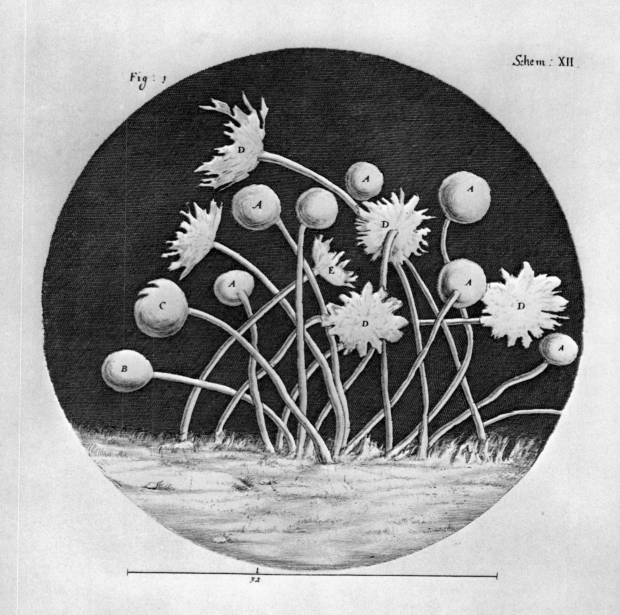

Fig: 1

Schem: XII

... a small white spot of hairy mould, multitudes of which I found to bespeck and whiten over the red covers of a small book. ... These spots appear'd, through a good microscope, to be a very pretty shap'd Vegetative body ... of small long cylindrical and transparent stalks ... with ... a round and white knob ... on the top of each ...; many of these knobs I observ'd to be very round, and of a smooth surface, such as AA, others smooth likewise, but a little oblong, as B; several of them a little broken or cloven with chops at the top, as C; others flitter'd as 'twere, or flown all to pieces, as DD.

5
Principles of Antimicrobial Therapy

The primary objective of antimicrobial therapy is eradication of the micro-organisms responsible for the infection. In many cases, this can be accomplished with a single course of therapy. In others, the infection will recur and require extended treatment.

SELECTION OF ANTIMICROBIAL AGENTS

The bacteria commonly associated with infection in the urinary tract vary widely in susceptibility to specific antimicrobial agents. As a rule, organisms responsible for acute infections in patients without previous urinary tract disease are more susceptible to antimicrobial drugs than organisms from patients with recurrent and complicated infections.[1] Some generalizations regarding their susceptibility to antimicrobial agents are shown in Figure 42.

Variations in susceptibility to antibacterial compounds make it impossible to predict with certainty the sensitivity of a specific bacterial isolate. For this reason, the use of antimicrobial susceptibility tests is essential in the selection of appropriate drugs for the treatment of urinary tract infections.

obert: Micrographia. London, 1665. (Courtesy of the Lilly Library, Indiana University, Bloomington, Indiana)

Figure 42. *Differences among gram-negative urinary pathogens in their susceptibility to selected antibiotics, as revealed by laboratory tests. The antibiotics listed with each group are those to which most strains are susceptible. The listings are not exhaustive. The percentages refer to acute infections (caused by the organisms listed) which occur in patients without obstruction who have not been treated with antimicrobial agents or subjected to urologic procedures.*

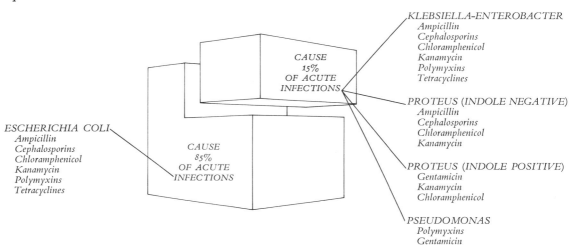

Figure 43. *Determination of the minimum inhibitory concentration by the broth-dilution method. The MIC in the example is 16 mcg./ml.*

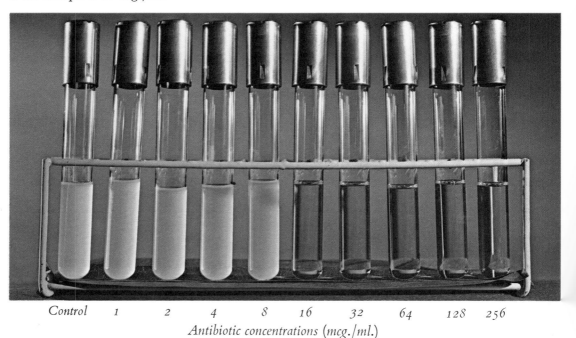

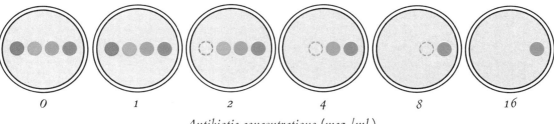

Antibiotic concentrations (mcg./ml.)

Figure 44. Determination of minimum inhibitory concentration by agar dilution. The antibiotic was diluted to give final concentrations as shown. The agar medium is indicated by the gray surface in the petri plates. Four different organisms were inoculated on each plate. The resulting colonies are represented symbolically by color. If the fate of each colony is followed, beginning with the plate of lowest antibiotic concentration, the first appearance of the dashed circle replacing the colony of the same color occurs at 2 mcg./ml. and indicates the lowest antibiotic concentration without growth; it is, therefore, the MIC for that culture. The MIC's for the two other cultures represented by the dashed circles are 4 and 8 mcg./ml. The fourth culture is resistant to the highest concentration of antibiotic in the test; hence, growth has occurred in all plates, and its MIC is not determined.

When the infection is asymptomatic or minimally symptomatic, as in the majority of cases, it is possible to await the results of susceptibility tests before beginning therapy. In occasional cases of acute pyelonephritis or of prostatitis, however, the systemic manifestations of infection may be severe and may be associated with bacteremia. In such patients, especially when bloodstream invasion is suspected, therapy must be initiated immediately, i.e., before the results of bacteriologic study and laboratory tests are available. (See section on Treatment of Sepsis, page 79.)

Determination of Susceptibility—The selection of an antibiotic for therapy of bacterial infections is dependent on knowledge of the susceptibility of the infecting organism. It is generally possible to determine susceptibility by in-vitro tests, which measure the antibiotic's ability to inhibit bacterial growth. The necessary tests may be done by either *dilution* or *diffusion* methods.

In dilution procedures, various concentrations of the antibiotic are made in broth or agar media, which are then inoculated with a standard number of the test organisms. The lowest antibiotic concentration which prevents growth after overnight incubation— the *minimum inhibitory concentration* (MIC)—is the measure of susceptibility. The appearance of the results in broth and agar tests is shown in Figures 43 and 44 respectively.

In diffusion test methods, paper discs are impregnated with the antibiotic and placed on agar uniformly seeded with the organism. A concentration gradient forms by diffusion of the antibiotic from the disc to inhibit growth of a sensitive organism. The basis for judging susceptibility may be the mere presence or absence of a zone without growth, as in the multiple-disc procedures in which a number of discs are used, each with a different amount of the antibiotic (Figure 45).

In the more convenient and reliable single-disc methods, only one disc is used for each antibiotic. A number of different antibiotics can be tested simultaneously, depending on

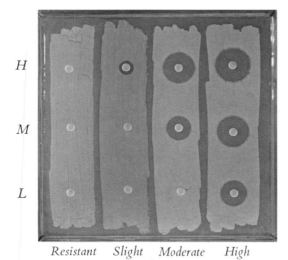

H

M

L

Resistant   Slight   Moderate   High

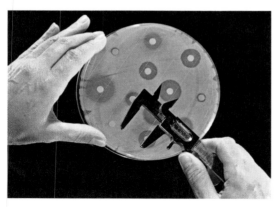

Figure 46. In single-disc susceptibility tests, the zone of inhibition is measured to the nearest millimeter.

the petri plate size. Each disc contains a specified amount of an antibiotic, and the criterion of susceptibility is the *actual size of the inhibition zone* measured to the nearest millimeter (Figure 46).

The size of the inhibition zone is *not* related in any simple way to degree of susceptibility. It is significantly influenced by the diffusion rate of the antibiotic outward from the discs into the agar, the type of culture medium, and the size of the bacterial inoculum. Thus, standardized procedures, such as the Bauer-Kirby[2] or the International Collaborative Study,[3] should be used if disc-diffusion methods are to be reliable aids in the selection of therapeutic agents.

Estimation of bacterial susceptibility by the disc test is qualitative or, at best, semiquantitative. Minimum inhibitory concentration values determined by broth or agar-dilution methods are considered more accurate estimates. Nevertheless, an important relationship exists between MIC data and inhibition zone diameters when these are determined according to a rigidly standardized procedure. This correlation is illustrated for an idealized situation in Figure 47. The "experimentally" determined points fall along a straight line, the "regression line."[4,5] Therefore, zone diameter is a *measure of MIC*, and the two are inversely related.

The correlation of minimum inhibitory concentrations with zone diameters (expressed in the regression line) is the basis for estimating bacterial susceptibility by the simple and rapidly performed disc-diffusion methods. (Because they are technically more complex—and hence more difficult to perform—dilution methods are not generally used in routine clinical work.)

Interpretation of Zone Sizes—To serve as guides for therapy, in-vitro tests (i.e., disc-diffusion methods performed according to a standardized procedure) must predict probable in-vivo effectiveness of the antimicrobial agents. The range of zone sizes for predictive purposes is the result of correlation of zone diameters with MIC values *in the light of clinical experience with the antibiotic. For pur-*

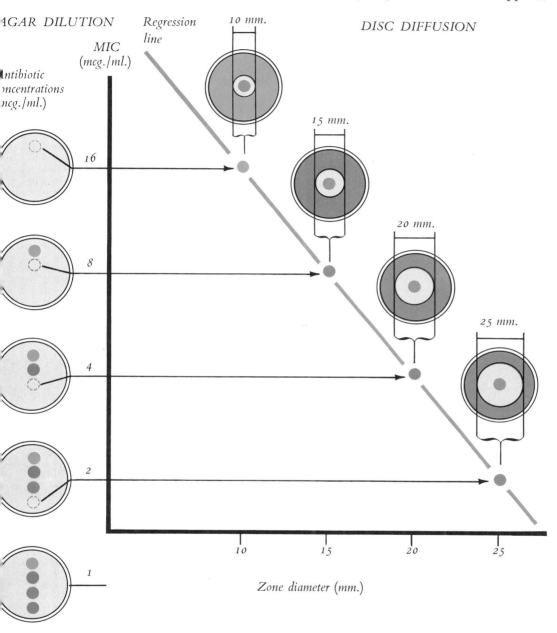

AGAR DILUTION

Regression line

DISC DIFFUSION

MIC (mcg./ml.)

Antibiotic oncentrations ncg./ml.)

10 mm.

15 mm.

20 mm.

25 mm.

16

8

4

2

1

10   15   20   25

Zone diameter (mm.)

Figure 47. Correlation of dilution and diffusion test data with four bacterial isolates. Each culture is represented a color, which appears as a colony (agar-dilution test) and as confluent growth (disc-diffusion test). The convention adopted for determination of MIC is that of Figure 44. In the diffusion test, the disc is blue and the inhibited zone is the gray area (the agar surface), and its diameter is indicated in millimeters. Beyond this zone, confluent growth is shown in the color representative for each organism. The blue line drawn through the plot of MIC vs. zone diameters is the regression line.

poses of interpretation, it is convenient to divide the zone sizes into three categories:

Resistant:	The organism is not likely to respond to therapy with the antibiotic.
Intermediate Susceptibility:	The organism is susceptible if dosage is high or if the antibiotic is concentrated in the urine.
Susceptible:	The organism is susceptible to ordinary dosage.

A list of some common antimicrobial agents with suggested interpretations of zone sizes determined according to the FDA disc method appears in Table 6.

Drug Safety and Efficacy—It must be emphasized that selection of an antibiotic for therapy cannot be based solely on the results of laboratory tests, because antibiotics of equal susceptibility in vitro may not be equally effective as therapeutic agents. In addition, knowledge of other characteristics of the antibiotics being considered and an estimation of their effect on the patient are required to make the best choice.

In this respect, the factor which demands the most careful appraisal is the drug's safety with regard to the patient. In general, if an organism is found to be approximately equal in susceptibility to several antibiotics, the drug of choice would probably be the one with the least serious toxic properties. This balance between safety and efficacy calls for a high degree of responsibility on the part of the prescribing physician.

The decision to administer drugs to pregnant women should be reached only after the potential hazard to both mother and fetus is carefully assessed. *The antibiotic used to treat a urinary tract infection during pregnancy sho[u]* *be one known to have no adverse effects on [the]* *fetus unless the susceptibility of the specific [in-]* *fecting organism makes such a choice impossi[ble.]*

BACTERIOLOGIC RESPONSES TO THERAPY

The physician needs to follow the therapeu[tic] response of his patient with repeated quan[ti-] tative urine cultures. A properly collect[ed] cleanly voided specimen of urine usually gi[ves] satisfactory results. Catheterization or blad[der] puncture to collect urine for routine cult[ure] is not required unless special circumstan[ces] (e.g., inability to co-operate) prevail (but [see] page 32). False-positive cultures are usua[lly] caused by contamination from an i[m]properly cleansed urethra or vulva or fr[om] improper handling of the sample after c[ol]lection. It should be emphasized that uri[ne] specimens must be cultured within a f[ew] minutes after collection or be plac[ed] promptly under refrigeration. If these pr[e]cautions are not observed, the small num[ber] of bacteria that are always present in voi[ded] specimens multiply rapidly and give fal[se] positive results.

Cure without Recurrence—Many patie[nts] with lower-urinary-tract infections or ac[ute] pyelonephritis who have neither a history [of] previous infection nor structural or functio[nal] abnormalities of the urinary tract will [re]spond rapidly, and without relapse or re[in]fection, to appropriate antimicrobial thera[py] (Figure 48a). Some patients recover sym[p]tomatically even in the absence of antibio[tic] therapy. Withholding antibiotics is not re[c]ommended, of course, but the existence [of] spontaneous cures does serve as evidence t[hat] symptomatic control of uncomplicated u[ri]nary tract infections may be relatively sim[ple] and successful.

Table 6

INTERPRETATIVE CHART OF ZONE SIZE
(FDA Standardized Disc Method)

Therapeutic Agent*	Test Disc†	Inhibition Zone Diameter (mm.)		
		Resistant	Intermediate Susceptibility	Suscep-tible
Cefazolin‡	Cephalothin, 30 mcg.	14 or less	15-17	18 or more
Cephalexin		14 or less	15-17	18 or more
Cephaloridine		14 or less	15-17	18 or more
Cephalothin		14 or less	15-17	18 or more
Cephaloglycin§		14 or less	—	15 or more
Chloramphenicol	30 mcg.	12 or less	13-17	18 or more
Gentamicin	10 mcg.	12 or less	—	13 or more
Kanamycin	30 mcg.	13 or less	14-17	18 or more
Nalidixic acid‡§	30 mcg.	13 or less	14-18	19 or more
Nitrofurantoin‡§	300 mcg.	14 or less	15-16	17 or more
Polymyxin B	300 units	8 or less	9-11	12 or more
Sulfonamides‡§	300 mcg.	12 or less	13-16	17 or more
Tetracyclines	Tetracycline, 30 mcg.	14 or less	15-18	19 or more
Ampicillin	10 mcg.			
Gram-negative organisms; enterococci		11 or less	12-13	14 or more
Staphylococci‖		20 or less	21-28	29 or more
Penicillin G	10 units			
Staphylococci		20 or less	21-28	29 or more
Other organisms		11 or less	12-21¶	22 or more

Listing adapted from Federal Register, *37*:20525, 1972, with exceptions as noted.

Structurally related antibiotics with similar activity spectra are tested against one member of the antibiotic family, as indicated. In the remaining examples listed, the antibiotic in the disc and the therapeutic agent are identical.

Not listed in Federal Register.

Urinary tract infections only.

Includes penicillin-G-susceptible organisms.

Includes organisms, such as enterococci and gram-negative bacilli, which may cause systemic infections treatable by high doses.

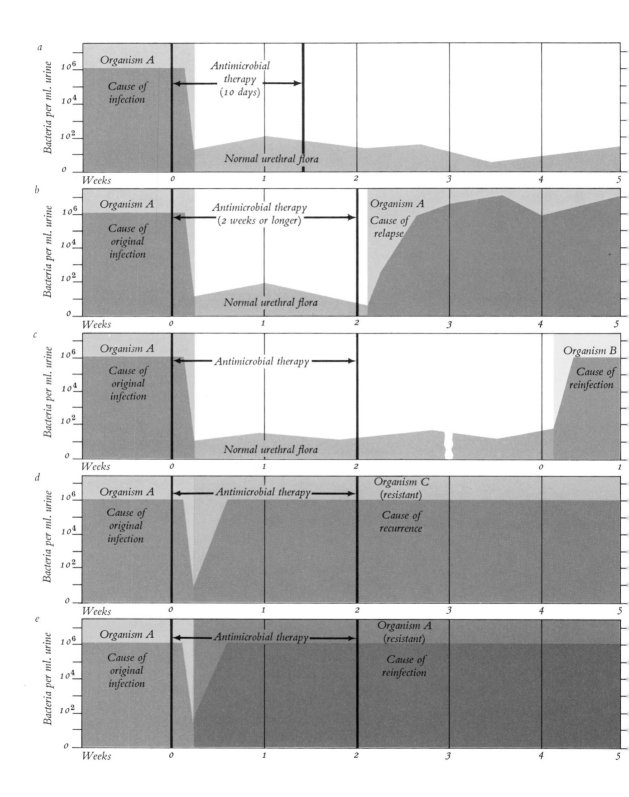

Figure 48. Types of bacteriologic responses to antimicrobial therapy. Background color appears during the time an infection is present, with the responsible organism indicated in each situation. The graph—in solid color in the foreground—shows the effect of therapy on the number of organisms per ml. of urine, i.e., on the bacteriologic course of the infection. Changes in color of the graphs emphasize the various responses which may occur after therapy is started. The normal flora is shown by portions of the graph in light blue.

a. Cure without recurrence.

b. Relapse after therapy. The organism which reappears is the same one that was present before therapy. Its susceptibility to the antibiotic has remained unchanged.

c. Reinfection. The initial organism (A) has been eliminated by antimicrobial therapy, but reinfection with another organism (B) has occurred. When reinfection is caused by the same species that produced the initial infection, it is difficult to differentiate it from relapse.

d. Infection with a different species or another serotype of the same species. The initial organism (A) is susceptible to the antibiotic in use, whereas the second organism (C) is resistant. Organism C may have been present in small numbers before therapy and emerged while the susceptible organism A was being eliminated; or organism C may represent reinfection which occurred during therapy.

e. Emergence of resistant mutant. The second organism is the same species and serologic type as the original, but it is resistant to the antimicrobial agent in use.

Relapse—On the other hand, clinical cure of chronic bacteriuria without recurrence takes place in only about one-fifth of patients after a single two-week course of antimicrobial therapy. In a large proportion of patients, *relapse* is due to the same organism that was present before therapy.[6] Although not detectable in the urine during therapy, the original organism may reappear in large numbers shortly after discontinuance of therapy (Figure 48b).

Reinfection—Recurrence of bacteriuria after therapy may be caused also by *reinfection* (Figures 48c and 48d).[6] It represents failure of host defense mechanisms to prevent bacterial invasion of the urinary bladder or failure to eliminate organisms that have gained access to the urinary tract. The common pattern in these patients is an apparently endless series of new infections which develop at variable times after each preceding organism has been successfully eradicated.

Mixed Infection—Some patients with chronic bacteriuria may have infection with multiple organisms ("mixed infection"). A single, or primary, organism usually predominates in the urine in high titer, whereas others—i.e., secondary organisms present in low titer—may not be detected on routine quantitative culture. However, if the organisms present in low titer are resistant to the antimicrobial agent in use, they may multiply as the antibiotic-susceptible primary organism is inhibited (Figure 48d).

Resistant Mutants—During antimicrobial therapy of both acute and chronic urinary tract infections, the antibiotic-susceptible bacteria may be replaced by antibiotic-resistant mutants (Figure 48e). When therapy is started, susceptible organisms are eliminated quickly; only the extremely small number which can resist the action of the antibiotic are then left to multiply. For this reason, the mutant, if it appears at all, will emerge very early. Although resistance may develop to any antimicrobial agent commonly used in urinary tract infections, it appears to occur more frequently with some than with others.

Urine Culture during Therapy—Under ideal circumstances, a quantitative urine culture should be obtained on the third or fourth day after antimicrobial therapy is begun. This is mandatory, of course, when clinical response is doubtful or slow. In the majority of cases, evidence of satisfactory bacteriologic response is apparent within a day or two. However, *prompt clinical improvement cannot be taken to indicate bacteriologic success*.[7] Generally, the organism initially isolated will not be recoverable from urine obtained after three to four days of successful therapy, and the quantitative culture will show fewer than 100,000 organisms per ml.

If, after this time, the urine culture is positive and the urine contains 100,000 or more organisms per ml., additional bacteriologic analysis is needed. The organism should be isolated from the culture and identified; laboratory tests should be performed and urine culture repeated to confirm the findings.

A positive culture with significant numbers of bacteria in the urine after the third or fourth day of therapy is usually caused by one of the following:

1. An organism initially present in the infection in small numbers, although resistant, could not greatly increase until the overwhelming population of the susceptible strain was reduced by the antibiotic.

2. Another organism capable of causing infection gained access to the urinary tract and, because of its resistance to the antimicrobial agent in use, proliferated and soon became dominant.

3. Resistant mutants of the original strain have been unaffected by the antibiotic and have increased in number.

4. The original laboratory tests were incorrect, and the organism is actually resistant to the drug being administered.

5. Antibiotic levels in the urine are ineffective because of insufficient dosage, poor absorption, or other factors.

Evaluation of Therapeutic Regimen—The presence of bacteria in large numbers in the urine three to four days after the start of therapy makes it necessary to reexamine the therapeutic regimen. If another organism (other than that initially believed responsible for the infection) or a resistant mutant (a variant of the original infecting organism) has appeared, the antimicrobial drug should be changed to one effective against both primary and secondary organisms. If such an agent is not available, the original therapy should be continued and additional drugs administered to control the secondary organism.

On the other hand, if the culture shows that the urine contains fewer than 100,000 bacteria per ml., it is likely that the therapy is effective and should be continued without interruption for a suitable period of time (see the following section). Urine culture should be prepared two to three weeks after treatment is stopped and again after six weeks and repeated three, six, and twelve months later.

Patients on long-term "suppressive" antimicrobial therapy because of persistent and recurrent infections should have cultures made at intervals of about one to three months to determine whether therapy is adequate. As a rule, symptomatic infection is preceded by the reappearance of bacteria in the urine. The appearance of organisms in large numbers is a warning signal that modification of therapy is needed. If appropriate changes are made, the recurrence of symptomatic disease may be effectively prevented.

DURATION OF THERAPY

Acute Infections—A course of therapy lasting ten days is often adequate in acute urinary tract infections treated with agents that are known to reach effective antibacterial levels both in tissues and in the urine. This period of treatment is sufficient to eradicate infection in about 85 percent of initial cases of acute lower-urinary-tract infections or acute pyelonephritis but is effective in only about 20 percent of patients with chronic infection, i.e., persistent or recurrent bacteriuria. Treatment over a period of two to three weeks should be considered in patients who suffer a relapse after the minimum ten days of therapy.[8]

Chronic Infections—When the infections are chronic, the type of antimicrobial agents selected for initial and long-term administration, the duration of therapy, and the number of therapeutic courses must be determined by weighing the potential severity of the infection against the potential inconveniences and/or toxicity of therapy. In certain patients —elderly women with asymptomatic infections, for example—it may sometimes be better to let the infection exist rather than proceed with repeated courses of anti-infective drugs. Decisions of this type can be made only after all aspects of each individual case have been considered.

TREATMENT OF SEPSIS

Patients with acute pyelonephritis occasionally develop bacteremia and manifestations of severe progressive systemic infection. As a rule, bacteremia with gram-negative bacilli requires prompt therapy. The over-all mortality rate is about 30 percent, with a high of 70 percent in patients who develop shock presumably due to the endotoxins of the infecting organism.[9]

To begin therapy in cases of gram-negative sepsis at the earliest possible moment is a departure from the practice followed under less pressing circumstances. Thus, administration of antimicrobial drugs should be initiated in these cases before the results of culture studies and laboratory tests are available.

Under these conditions, successful management depends on selection of agents with the widest possible range of antimicrobial activity. A single drug may not be satisfactory under all circumstances, even when the infection is caused by any of the organisms usually encountered. To obtain the needed antibacterial activity against almost all of the enteric gram-negative bacilli that might be responsible for bacteremia secondary to urinary tract infection, it may be necessary to use several drugs in combination.[10] Drug therapy can be modified later in accordance with the results of culture studies and susceptibility tests. The duration of treatment with systemically active antimicrobial agents should be at least ten days to two weeks. In addition, supportive measures are usually required.

PHARMACOLOGIC CONSIDERATIONS

Bactericidal versus Bacteriostatic Antibiotics—The effectiveness of *bactericidal antibiotics*—those that kill—as compared with *bacteriostatic antibiotics*—those that inhibit multiplication—has been the subject of considerable discussion and controversy. Although it would appear theoretically advantageous to kill rather than to inhibit the infecting organisms, such advantage is not substantiated by data now available. Urinary tract infections often respond satisfactorily to agents that simply inhibit bacterial multiplication. It must be remembered that recovery from infection no doubt results from antimicrobial drug action in conjunction with the normal defense mechanism of the host.

Effective Antibiotic Levels— To achieve optimum therapy in urinary tract infections, either bactericidal or bacteriostatic concentrations of antibiotic are required wherever organisms are multiplying. Effective amounts of antibiotic must be present in the interstitial tissues of the renal parenchyma, in the urine during the time it is in any part of the urinary system, or in both sites. When the appropriate level of antibiotic is maintained, the antimicrobial property of the drug is fully utilized to aid the host's defenses in destroying the cause of infection.

Significance of High Antibiotic Levels in the Urine—Some antimicrobial agents are not retained for any significant length of time in the blood or tissues. Instead, they appear to be concentrated in the renal tubules or, in some cases, to be converted to an active form during passage through the kidney. In any case, the urine contains therapeutic levels, often quite high, whereas blood and tissues do not. For this reason, the effectiveness of such drugs is greatest in lower-urinary-tract infections when the renal parenchyma is not involved.

Undoubtedly, since the site of infection in the vast majority of patients with bacteriuria is confined to the bladder without any spread to the kidney, it is not surprising that effective therapy is obtained with these agents.

Even when the renal parenchyma is infected, drugs having maximum activity in the urine may, nevertheless, be useful therapeutically. It should be recalled that the kidney is most likely to be reinfected by bacteria which are growing and multiplying in the urine. In this manner, kidney infection is perpetuated despite the tendency of the host's defense mechanisms to eradicate the invading organism. Removal of this reservoir of infecting organisms is a necessary step for elimination of infection within the kidney. Indeed, in the opinion of some authorities, if reinfection of the parenchyma did not occur, many patients with pyelonephritis would undergo spontaneous cure.

Consequently, the effectiveness of such agents in pyelonephritis lies in their ability to sterilize the urine and thereby eliminate the supply of pathogenic bacteria at the source. When this occurs, the infection remaining in the kidney is likely to be within the capabilities of the host's defense mechanism. Generally, these antimicrobial agents must be administered for long periods to allow natural processes sufficient time to remove bacteria from the sites of infection in the kidney.

BIBLIOGRAPHY

1. Lindemeyer, R. I., Turck, M., and Petersdorf, R. G.: Factors Determining the Outcome of Chemotherapy in Infections of the Urinary Tract, Ann. Int. Med., *58:*201, 1963.

2. Bauer, A. W., Kirby, W. M. M., Sherris, J. C., and Turck, M.: Antibiotic Susceptibility Testing by a Standardized Single Disk Method, Am. J. Clin. Path., 45:493, 1966.

3. WHO Expert Committee on Antibiotics: Second Report. Standardization of Methods for Conducting Microbic Sensitivity Tests, WHO Technical Report Series No. 210, 1961.

4. Ericsson, H.: The Disc Method in Quantitative Determination of Sensitivity to Antibiotics, Postgrad. M. J., *43* (Supplement):46, 1967.

5. Wick, W. E.: Delineation of the Differences of Various Bacterial Susceptibility Tests with Cephalexin, Antimicrob. Agents & Chemother., p. 435, 1968.

6. Turck, M., Anderson, K. N., and Petersdorf, R. G.: Relapse and Reinfection in Chronic Bacteriuria, New England J. Med., *275:*70, 1966.

7. Freedman, L. R.: Pyelonephritis and Urinary Tract Infection, in Diseases of the Kidney (edited by M. B. Strauss and L. G. Welt), p. 469. Boston: Little, Brown & Company, 1963.

8. Kincaid-Smith, P., and Fairley, K. F.: Controlled Trial Comparing Effect of Two and Six Weeks' Treatment in Recurrent Urinary Tract Infection, Brit. M. J., *2:*145, 1969.

9. Maiztegui, J. I., Biegeleisen, J. Z., Jr., Cherry, W. B., and Kass, E. H.: Bacteremia Due to Gram-Negative Rods; A Clinical, Bacteriologic, Seriologic and Immunofluorescent Study, New England J. Med., *272:* 222, 1965.

10. The Medical Letter on Drugs and Therapeutics, Issue 254, October 4, 1968.

GENERAL REFERENCES

Bengtsson, U., Lincoln, K., and Hood, B.: Long-term Antibacterial Treatment of Chronic Pyelonephritis, Acta med. scandinav., *181:*641, 1967.

Brumfitt, W., and Percival, A.: Adjustment of Urine pH in the Chemotherapy of Urinary-Tract Infections, Lancet, *1:*186, 1962.

Gutman, L. T., Turck, M., Petersdorf, R. G., and Wedgwood, R. J.: Significance of Bacterial Variants in Urine of Patients with Chronic Bacteriuria, J. Clin. Invest., *44:*1945, 1965.

Guze, L. B., and Kalmanson, G. M.: Persistence of Bacteria in "Protoplast" Form after Apparent Cure of Pyelonephritis in Rats, Science, *143:*1340, 1964.

Kunin, C. M.: A Guide to Use of Antibiotics in Patients with Renal Disease, Ann. Int. Med., *67:*151, 1967.

McCabe, W. R., and Jackson, G. G.: Treatment of Pyelonephritis: Bacterial, Drug and Host Factors in Success or Failure among 252 Patients, New England J. Med., *272:*1037, 1965.

Stamey, T. A., Govan, D. E., and Palmer, J. M.: The Localization and Treatment of Urinary Tract Infections: The Role of Bactericidal Urine Levels as Opposed to Serum Levels, Medicine, *44:*1, 1965.

Turck, M., Ronald, A. R., and Petersdorf, R. G.: Relapse and Reinfection in Chronic Bacteriuria. II. The Correlation between Site of Infection and Pattern of Recurrence in Chronic Bacteriuria, New England J. Med., *278:*422, 1968.

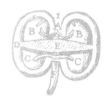
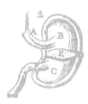

DE VISCERVM
STRVCTVRA
EXERCITATIO
ANATOMICA
MARCELLI MALPIGHII

Philoſ. & Med. Bononien. in Meſſa-
nenſi Academia Medicinę
Primarij.

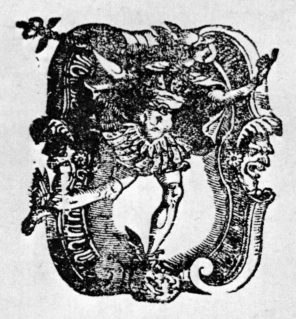

BONONIÆ,

Ex Typographia Iacobi Montij. MDCLXVI.
Superiorum permiſſu.

R. C.

6

Structures and Functions of the Kidney

Knowledge of the kidney's structure and its role in health is essential to an understanding of the effects of infection and the patient's therapeutic needs during the clinical course of his disease.

INTRODUCTION

The Nephron—The functions of the kidney are carried out by nephrons. There are about one million in each kidney, arranged in radially positioned, parallel rows. (The structures in a kidney lobe and their relationships are represented in three dimensions in Figure 49. A nephron and related components are shown diagrammatically in Figure 59, page 104. For the description which follows, reference may be made to either illustration.) The nephron consists of Bowman's capsule, which surrounds a network of capillaries, called the "capillary, or glomerular, tuft" or simply the "glomerulus." Tuft and capsule together are the Malpighian body, or renal corpuscle. The capsule is attached to a tubule composed of a proximal portion, Henle's loop, a distal portion, and a collecting duct.

The renal corpuscle and the distal and proximal convoluted tubules are confined to the cortical portion of the kidney. Here, too, is the juxtaglomerular apparatus (JGA), a component in the hormonal control of kidney function. Throughout the cortical region,

Figure 49. Schematic relationship of structures in a renal pyramid. The direction of view is down a collecting duct and toward the kidney pelvis.

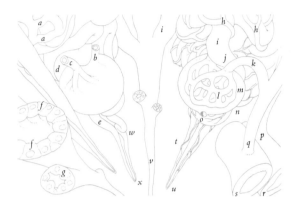

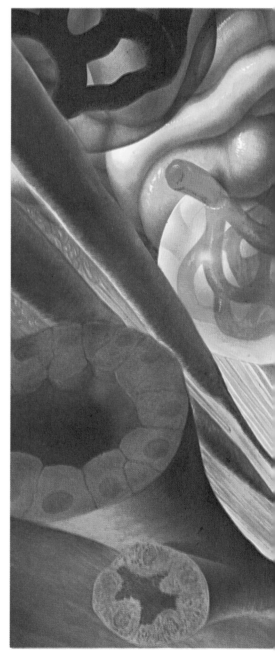

a. Peritubular capillaries

b. Efferent arteriole

c. Afferent arteriole

d. Distal convolutions

e. Ascending limb

f. Collecting duct

g. Distal convolutions joining collecting duct

h. Peritubular capillaries

i. Distal convolutions

j. Region of the juxtaglomerular apparatus

k. Afferent arteriole

l. Glomerulus

m. Bowman's space

n. Bowman's capsule

o. Proximal convolutions

p. Interlobular vein

q. Interlobular artery

r. Arcuate vein

s. Arcuate artery

t. Vasa recta

u. Henle's loop

v. Collecting duct

w. Descending limb

x. Thin portion of Henle's loop

the vascular system resembles a plexus that accommodates perhaps 90 percent of the blood reaching the kidney.

Henle's loop and the major portion of each collecting duct are found in the renal medulla. The salt gradient of the medullary

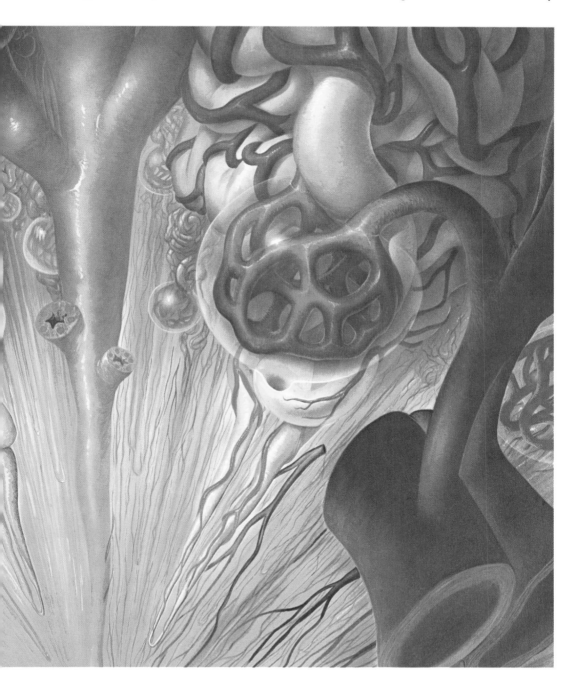

Figure 50. Diagrammatic representation of tubular functions. Filtration occurs in the renal corpuscle, which is represented by the cup-shaped structure. The filtrate is shown in yellow. Each function is indicated by an arrow pointing in an appropriate direction and located either proximally or distally along the tubule. The color of the arrow represents the specific substance undergoing the functions shown.

a. Filtration and excretion, as with inulin.

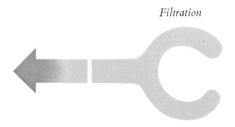

b. Filtration and reabsorption *(proximally)*, as with glucose.

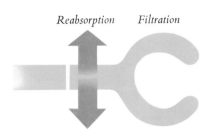

c. Filtration and secretion *(proximally)*, as with p-aminohippuric acid.

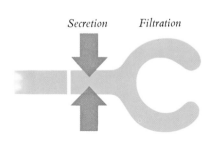

d. Filtration, reabsorption *(proximally)*, and secretion *(distally)*, as with potassium ions.

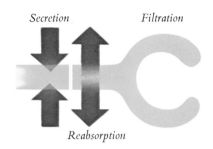

interstitium is an essential component of the urine-concentrating mechanism. Accordingly, a special system, the *vasa recta*, is needed to supply blood without destroying this gradient.

Operations of the Nephron—In essence, a nephron is a tube which contains a virtually protein-free filtrate of plasma at one end and delivers urine at its opposite end. The numerous and complex events required to bring about this transformation begin in the renal corpuscle, where the glomerular capillaries' unique structure permits them to function as bulk filters. The resulting glomerular fluid immediately begins to undergo changes which continue until it is excreted as urine.

Not all substances that make up glomerular fluid are treated in the same way. Some components of the glomerular filtrate simply pass down the tubules and out of the kidneys without alteration in amount, as with inulin (Figure 50a). Except for back-diffusion, this description probably applies also to urea. Other substances are actively reabsorbed (Figure 50b). The degree of reabsorption may be almost complete (as with glucose and amino acids) or variable (as with water and ions). Variability in reabsorption is frequently dependent on hormonal action. For instance, reabsorption of water from the collecting duct, which produces an appropriately concentrated urine, is regulated by hormonally controlled adjustments of the duct's permeability.

Secretion also occurs in the tubules (Figure 50c). In this way, various organic cations and anions as well as potassium, ammonium, and hydrogen ions are added to tubular contents. Some substances undergo both reabsorption and secretion, although in different portions of the tubule (Figure 50d).

Since the fundamental operations of filtration, reabsorption, and secretion are integrated in health, the kidneys carry out the following essential functions:

1. Regulation of volume and composition of body fluids, i.e.,
   a. Conservation of water and essential substances
   b. Maintenance of acid-base balance
2. Detoxification and excretion of noxious, foreign, or nonessential materials

The mechanisms and interrelationships of these vital activities in health will be considered in the ensuing pages.

PRODUCTION OF GLOMERULAR FLUID

Glomerular fluid is produced by a process of filtration in the glomerular capillaries, which differ from other capillaries in several important ways. They are unique in that they are placed between two arterioles rather than between an arteriole and a venule. The arterioles are of dissimilar size. The *afferent* arteriole that brings blood to the tuft is larger in diameter than is the *efferent* arteriole that drains the tuft. This arrangement, plus a mechanism to change the size of the arterioles as conditions require, is believed to account for the unusually high hydrostatic pressure in the glomerular capillaries. Finally, they differ in structure from other capillaries, and their permeability is appreciably greater. The essential features of glomerular capillaries and related structures appear in Figure 51.

Glomerular Hydrostatic Pressure—Hydrostatic, or "blood," pressure is produced by contraction of the heart and is responsible for supplying the energy for filtration in all the capillaries of the body. In the glomerulus, it is equivalent to 75 mm. Hg, approximately

Figure 51. Schematic representation from electron micrographs of a three-dimensional section through a renal corpuscle.

The outermost structure of the renal corpuscle is Bowman's capsule, which consists of a parietal layer of epithelium (shown only as part of a cell and nucleus) and—separated by the urinary, or Bowman's, space—a visceral epithelial layer. The visceral epithelium is also the outer covering of the glomerular capillaries, which contain, in addition, a central basement membrane and an inner endothelial layer. The capillary loops—four are shown—that make up the glomerulus are arranged around the centrally placed irregular mesangial cells.

Much of the cytoplasm of each endothelial cell in the lining of the capillary loops resembles a thin sheet, as though the cell had been stretched out to cover a large area. In this attenuated part are numerous fenestrations that superficially resemble holes, or pores; actually, each is covered by a thin diaphragm with a central knob as represented in a.

The basement membrane may be composed of several layers but is considered to be continuous; i.e., it contains

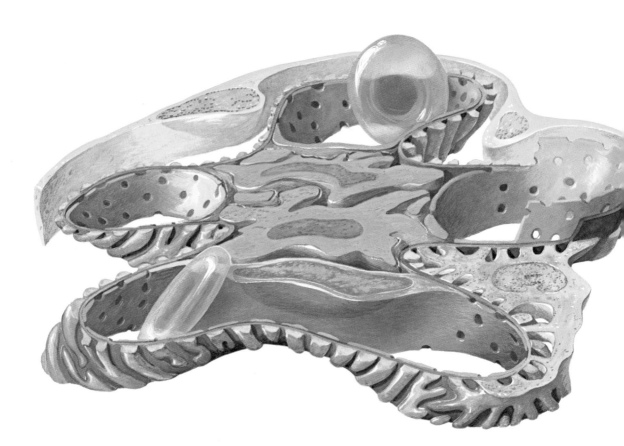

holes. It may consist of fibrils embedded in a mucopolysaccharide matrix and thus, as suggested by some, may semble a gel both in structure and in mode of action.

The characteristic structural features of the cells that form the epithelial layer are the podocytes, long ten- clelike cell extensions, and numerous footlike structures, the pedicels, which arise from them. A pedicel literally stands" in the basement membrane on a "foot" that is broader than the remainder of the structure. The ar- ngement of the pedicels leaves some space between them, which creates the so-called "slit pores." Slit pores e also formed when the pedicels interlock with similar structures from the same or neighboring cells. In either se, the "pore" is covered with a membrane which is reinforced by a slight thickening along its center, as in b.

The fine structure of the glomerular capillaries suggests that filtration requires passage of material through ree filtration barriers—the membrane covering of the endothelial fenestrations, the basement membrane itself, d the slit membrane in the epithelium. Inasmuch as no true holes exist in the capillary wall, selectivity may e the function of each filtration barrier, individually or in consort.

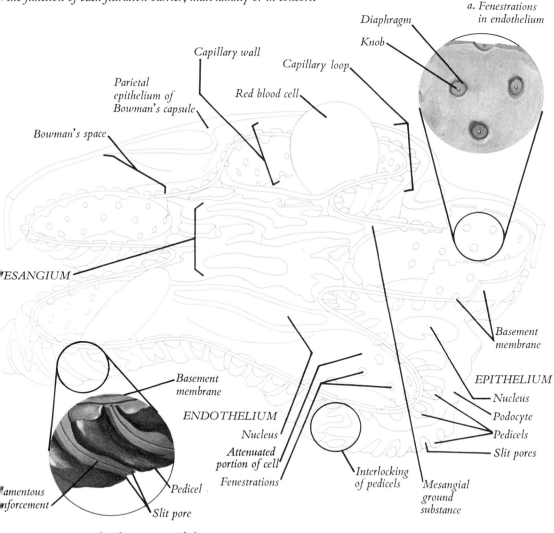

b. Slit pore in epithelium

Figure 52. The normal forces in glomerular filtration. Each large arrow represents the direction of the fo
either promoting or opposing filtration; the number indicates its magnitude.

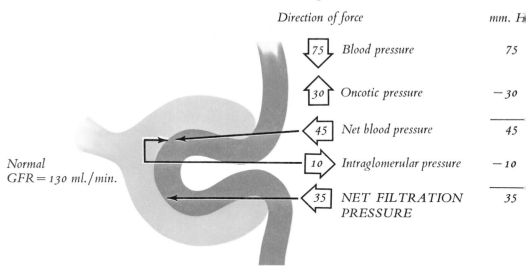

Direction of force	mm. H
Blood pressure	75
Oncotic pressure	−30
Net blood pressure	45
Intraglomerular pressure	−10
NET FILTRATION PRESSURE	35

Normal
GFR = 130 ml./min.

twice the pressure in other capillaries (Figure 52). It is maintained at this level during normal kidney function because resistance between afferent and efferent arterioles is kept in balance. When the afferent arteriole is constricted (with no change in renal artery pressure), filtration pressure drops. Constriction of the efferent arteriole produces the opposite effect—i.e., filtration pressure rises. The required variations in arteriolar size occur in small increments, so that large pressure fluctuations in the intervening capillary tuft are avoided.

The same mechanism prevents variations in blood pressure from affecting filtration pressure and filtration rate. Therefore, a decrease (within limits) in renal arterial pressure is compensated by dilatation of the afferent and constriction of the efferent arteriole.

Adjustment of arteriolar size is, in part, under the control of the renal nerves and is probably their major role. However, even when all nerve connections are severed, the kidney continues to maintain a remarkably constant blood flow and filtration rate inde-

pendent of fluctuations in renal arterial pre
sure. This unique method of pressure cont
is called "autoregulation" and appears to
a direct response by the arterioles to the pr
sure distending their walls.

***Osmotic Pressure of Plasma Proteins*—**T
osmotic pressure due to plasma proteins (t
oncotic pressure) opposes filtration pressu
that is, it tends to "keep fluid in" (Figure 5.
This pressure is equal to about 30 mm. F
and exists because large molecules in plasm
such as proteins, cannot pass through t
glomerular filter (Figure 53). According
the concentration of protein in glomerul
filtrate is negligible. In contrast, small mo
cules, such as plasma electrolytes, pass free
through the glomerular wall. Hence, th
concentration is approximately equal
plasma and filtrate. The slight difference is
consequence of the Donnan equilibrium; i.
anionic plasma proteins enhance efflux of f
trable anions and limit efflux of filtrable ca
ions. The concentration of anions is therefo
about 5 percent higher and the concentratio

*gure 53. Virtually all plasma proteins (large pur-
e discs) are retained by the glomerular filters, whereas
her substances, represented by the variously colored
aller discs, pass through. Hence, glomerular fluid
essentially a protein-free filtrate.*

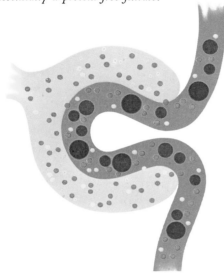

cations about 5 percent lower in glomer-
ar filtrate than in plasma.

Plasma osmotic pressure may affect filtra-
on under certain conditions. When glomer-
ar hydrostatic pressure is abnormally low,
e plasma osmotic pressure tends to diminish
rther the already reduced filtration. Con-
rsely, when the plasma osmotic pressure is
w (due to low plasma-protein concentra-
on, as in nephrotic syndrome), filtration
nds to increase.

traglomerular Hydrostatic Pressure—
he effect of hydrostatic pressure on filtration
opposed by the pressure of the fluid in
owman's space, i.e., the space between
owman's capsule and the glomerulus which
surrounds. The intraglomerular pressure or
tracapsular tissue pressure is equal to about
mm. Hg (Figure 52). It remains constant
nder normal conditions, but, in certain
athological states, changes occur that have

important effects on filtration. When there is
hindrance to urine outflow due, for example,
to obstruction of the ureter by renal calculus,
neoplasm, or prostatic hypertrophy, urine
"backs up" into the kidney (hydronephrosis)
and causes an increase in intraglomerular
pressure. Such pressure counteracts the force
favoring filtration.

Area and Porosity of Filtering Surface—
Filtration is influenced by the area and permeability of the filtering surface. Several factors appear to be important—the number of
glomeruli which are functionally active, the
total filtering area of these glomeruli, and the
fraction of the capillary tuft in each glomerulus which participates in the filtration process. The consensus is that all glomeruli in
healthy mammals are continuously active.
However, it is not clear whether all parts of
the capillary network in each glomerulus
function as filters with identical efficiency.

*Glomerular Filtration Rate—*From the preceding discussion it is obvious that some
forces promote filtration, whereas others
hinder it. In health, these forces are properly
balanced so that glomerular filtration keeps
pace with body requirements; in disease, that
may not occur. For this reason, the rate of
glomerular filtration is an important indica-
tor of renal function, and its measurement is
of considerable practical as well as theoretical
significance.

*Determination of Filtration Rate—*Determination of filtration rate requires use of
some substance that passes freely through the
glomeruli and is neither reabsorbed nor secreted by the tubules. That is, a substance is
needed which is subjected to only one of the
nephron's basic operations—filtration—and
is then excreted in the urine.

One such substance is inulin, a polysaccharide consisting of fructose units, which is derived from Jerusalem artichokes and dahlia tubers. It is a large molecule with a molecular weight said to be 5,200. It probably is a mixture of various-sized polymers. The measurement of glomerular filtration rate is based on considerations which may be conveniently

discussed with inulin as the test substance

The plasma components which pass freely through the glomerular filter have equal concentrations in plasma and filtrate. The concentration of inulin in plasma and filtrate is the same within a short time after its administration by intravenous injection. Therefore if the inulin concentration in plasma is found

---

BOX 3

THE EQUATION FOR GLOMERULAR FILTRATION RATE

The glomerular filtration rate (GFR) is given by:

$$GFR = K_p \left[(P_b - P_c) - \pi_b \right]$$

The symbols are defined in the accompanying tabulation.

Symbol	Force	Function
P_b	Hydrostatic pressure *of blood in glomerulus*	*Main driving force of filtration* (≈ 75 mm. Hg)
P_c	Hydrostatic pressure *of fluid in* Bowman's capsule	*Opposes filtration* (≈ 10 mm. Hg)
π_b	Osmotic pressure *of blood due to* plasma proteins (oncotic pressure)	*Opposes filtration* (≈ 30 mm. Hg)
K_p	Filtration permeability	*Relates porosity and area of filter surface to filtration*

The following statements arise from the equation:

—When the hydrostatic pressure in the glomerular tuft (P_b) increases, the filtration rate (GFR) also increases (a); a decrease in P_b results in a decrease in GFR (b).

—If decrease in P_b is marked, as might occur during shock, filtration may cease entirely and result in anuria (c). When the approximate numerical value as given above is substituted for each term in the equation, it is seen that GFR = 0 (filtration ceases) when P_b = 40 mm. Hg.

—An increase in hydrostatic pressure in Bowman's space (P_c) or an increase in osmotic pressure of plasma proteins (π_b) tends to decrease net filtration pressure and so to diminish filtration rate.

—A decrease in plasma protein osmotic pressure (π_b) tends to increase net filtration pressure and hence filtration rate.

by analysis to be 1 mg. per ml., the glomerular fluid also contains 1 mg. per ml.

The amount of any component in glomerular filtrate will remain unchanged during passage in the tubules when it is not reabsorbed, secreted, or capable of being diffused. However, because of change in water volume, its concentration does not remain constant.

The amount of inulin excreted in urine is the amount which was filtered in the glomeruli. Assuming that 1,000 mg. of inulin are found in a urine sample (and no loss or gain of inulin occurred in the tubules), the quantity excreted in the urine (1,000 mg.) is the exact amount that was filtered. If the plasma concentration is 1 mg. per ml., it would take

---

BOX 3 (Continued)

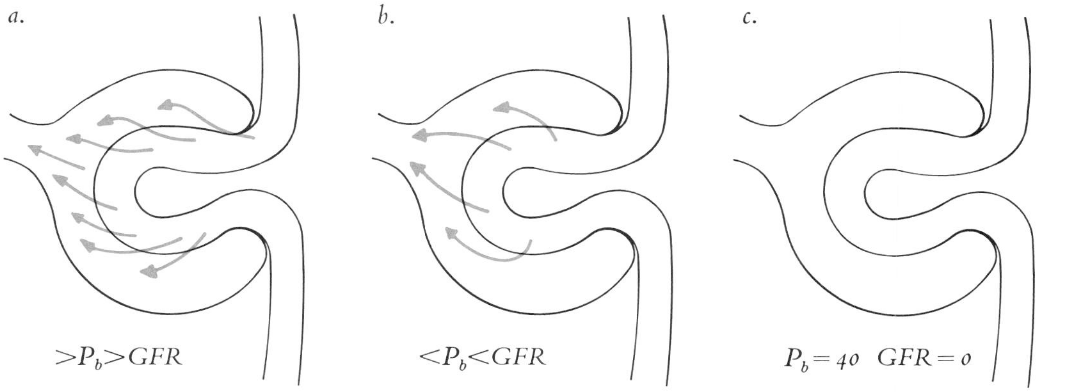

a.

$>P_b>GFR$

b.

$<P_b<GFR$

c.

$P_b=40 \quad GFR=0$

— *The equation contains no terms representing blood flow because, within broad limits in health, glomerular filtration is not dependent upon the amount of blood which passes through the glomerular capillaries. Thus, fluctuations in cardiac output, either above or below normal, need not produce corresponding changes in filtration rate as long as arterial pressure is maintained. However, flow rate may affect filtration rate indirectly. When the flow of blood through the glomerulus is abnormally. slow, time is available for each unit volume of plasma to lose more than the usual amount of its fluid by filtration and thereby become enriched in protein. One might say "the soup thickens," because the proteins are retained, whereas almost all other substances, including water, pass through the glomerular wall. As the protein concentration increases, plasma osmotic pressure also rises. In essence, filtration is hampered because fluids are retained, with the result that glomerular filtration rate diminishes. The opposite effect would occur if the flow of blood through the glomerulus were rapid. (The equation for GFR takes into account the effect of osmotic pressure without regard to any of the factors that may change its magnitude.)*

— *The effect of area and porosity of the filter enters into the term "K_p." However, K_p is not a biological constant.*

BOX 4

CALCULATION OF GFR

To obtain reliable data for calculation of glomerular filtration rate, urine must be collected at precise intervals. Furthermore, the inulin concentration in both plasma and urine must be measured. Without discussion of these technics or the rather complicated procedure for inulin determination, the following is illustrative of data obtained for a normal adult male:

Concentration of inulin in plasma (P_{IN})—*This was measured during the period of collection of urine and determined by analysis to be 0.2 mg. inulin per ml. plasma.*

Rate of urine flow (V)—*The volume of urine excreted during a specified period of time averaged 1 ml. per minute.*

Concentration of inulin in urine (U_{IN})—*The urine was found to contain 26 mg. inulin per ml.*

If these statements are used in two equations, the necessary calculations of the data can be made in a stepwise fashion. The rate of inulin excretion in the urine is determined in Equation 1. This result is used in Equation 2 for calculation of glomerular filtration rate.

Equation 1

Urinary excretion rate of inulin	=	Concentration of inulin in urine	·	Rate of urine flow
E_{IN}	=	U_{IN}	·	V

Rearranging and indicating units:

$$E_{IN} = U_{IN} \frac{(mg.\ inulin)}{(ml.\ urine)} \cdot V \frac{(ml.\ urine)}{(min.)}$$

$$E_{IN} = U_{IN}V \frac{(mg.\ inulin)}{(min.)}$$

When $U_{IN} = 26$ mg. per ml. and $V = 1$ ml. per minute, substitution of these data into Equation 1 gives:

$$U_{IN}V = \frac{26\ mg./ml.}{1\ ml./min.} = 26\ mg./min.$$

Conclusion: 26 ml. of inulin are excreted during each minute of urine flow.

---

filtration of 1,000 ml. of plasma to excrete this amount of inulin.

For determination of rate, one additional factor—time—must be considered. Accordingly, it is necessary to measure the amount of inulin excreted during a known time interval. In the above example, assume 1,000 mg.

of inulin were excreted during ten minutes of urine flow; urinary excretion is then 1,000 mg. per ten minutes or 100 mg. per minute. Inasmuch as plasma concentration is 1 mg. per ml., excretion of 100 mg. per minute requires the production of 100 ml. of glomerular fluid per minute. In other words, 100

BOX 4 (*Continued*)

When the rate of excretion of inulin in urine and its concentration in plasma are known, then the volume of fluid which must pass through the glomerular filter each minute—i.e., the glomerular filtration rate—is given by Equation 2.

Equation 2

$$\text{Glomerular filtration rate} = \frac{\text{Urinary excretion rate of inulin}}{\text{Concentration of inulin in plasma}}$$

$$GFR = \frac{U_{IN}V}{P_{IN}}$$

Rearranging and indicating units:

$$GFR = \frac{U_{IN}V \ (mg. \ inulin/min.)}{P_{IN} \ (mg. \ inulin/ml. \ plasma)}$$

$$GFR = U_{IN}V \cdot \frac{1 \ (mg. \ inulin)}{P_{IN} \ (min.)} \cdot \frac{(ml. \ plasma)}{(mg. \ inulin)}$$

$$GFR = \frac{U_{IN}V \ (ml. \ plasma)}{P_{IN} \ (min.)}$$

When $U_{IN}V = 26$ mg./min. and $P_{IN} = 0.2$ mg./ml., then:

$$GFR = \frac{26 \ mg./min.}{0.2 \ mg./ml.} = \frac{26 \ ml.}{0.2 \ min.} = 130 \ ml./min.$$

Conclusion: In this example, a normal adult male with two kidneys containing approximately 2,000,000 glomeruli produced 130 ml. of filtrate each minute.

---

ml. of fluid must pass through the glomerular filter each minute, or glomerular filtration rate (GFR) = 100 ml. per minute.

The Clearance Concept—It should be recalled that since the process of filtration does not change the concentration of inulin (or of any other substance which passes freely through the filter), plasma and glomerular fluid have similar inulin concentrations. Furthermore, the amount of inulin remains constant during its entire sojourn in the urinary tract; no change in quantity occurs from the time it is filtered until it is excreted.

Accordingly, the figure so obtained is *the volume of plasma which must have been filtered through the glomerular capillaries each minute to supply the amount of inulin found excreted in the urine.* The figure, however, is fictitious because it represents the volume of plasma needed each minute *as though* its entire content of inulin were filtered out—i.e., as though the plasma were "cleared" of inulin in a single journey through the glomerular capillaries (Figure 54).

The volume indicated by this "clearance" figure is described as a virtual volume (or volume *in effect*) to distinguish it from the

Figure 54. Inulin clearance is the volume of plasma needed each minute (represented in the figure to the left by the section of glomerular capillary between the white lines) as though the entire content of inulin were filtered out (right), i.e., as though the plasma had been "cleared" of inulin.

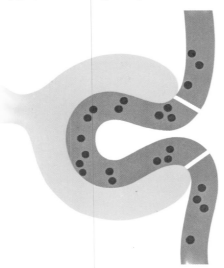 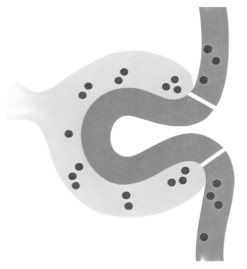

real (or *actual*) volume it purports to represent. However, the distinction between real and virtual volumes is without significance either for determination or interpretation of clearance. The clearance figure will have the same numerical value whether one unit of volume of plasma gives up one-half of its inulin content or two units of volume give up one-fourth of their inulin content.

Significance of Clearance Data—In health, the glomerular filtration rate is remarkably constant. The average inulin clearance in normal men is 125 ml. per minute per 1.73 square meters and approximately 10 percent less in women—115 ml. per minute per 1.73 square meters. (For purposes of comparison, inulin clearance data are corrected to a normal standard body surface area of 1.73 square meters.) Therefore, it can be calculated that the total volume of fluid which passes through the glomeruli in a twenty-four-hour period is 180 liters in men and 166 liters in women. Dissimilar size of the sexes does not account

for the difference in clearance, inasmuch as it persists after correction to the normal standard body surface area, as the above figures indicate.

In addition to determining filtration rate, the measurement of inulin clearance is a useful reference in studying the behavior of other substances in the tubules. Briefly, if a test substance is cleared in greater amount than inulin, the excess was added in the tubules; the test substance, unlike inulin, undergoes *tubular secretion*. If, however, clearance is less than with inulin, the opposite has occurred; that is, there has been a loss of the test substance in the tubule due to *tubular reabsorption*. If the clearance is the same as that of inulin, it may be assumed that the test substance is neither secreted nor absorbed and therefore behaves in the tubule like inulin.

Other Test Compounds—Although other substances are used to measure glomerular filtration rate, none is as good in a quantitative sense as inulin, and none is so suitable for etermining the effects of tubular action on a unknown substance. The most common f these inulin substitutes is creatinine. Its earance approximates the value for inulin, at this is the result of fortuitous circumstances. Creatinine is weakly secreted by the nal tubules. The resulting higher urinary xcretion is countered by substances in the lasma (and not present in urine) which enance the color reaction for creatinine. Thus, ecause of tubular secretion, the greater mount present in urine is balanced by the reater amount in plasma due to nonspecific olor reactions. The net result is a clearance pproximating that of inulin.

In disease states, creatinine clearance may ot agree with inulin clearance. This may be ue to creatinine-like chromogens in plasma r to enhanced permeability to creatinine exibited by cells lining the nephron. In spite of is limitation, creatinine is widely used to etermine glomerular filtration rates.

The endogenous creatinine clearance ethod is convenient because it does not reuire intravenous administration of a test ibstance (creatinine is a normal constituent f extracellular fluid), and analysis for creatine is technically simple.

Urea has frequently been employed to measure filtration rate, but its use has serious rawbacks. Because it diffuses slowly into ells, its excretion depends on its rate of flow. hus, reduced urine flow enhances diffusion to the tubular cells and makes clearance eceptively low. (Mathematical formulas are vailable to help correct such data.)

Other substances that have found limited se are mannitol and allantoin. Recently, idioactive vitamin B_{12} administered in a ngle injection has been recommended and nay give results as accurate as those with iulin without the technical difficulties of iulin infusion and chemical determination.

TUBULAR REABSORPTION AND SECRETION

If we recall the magnitude of glomerular filtration, we can better appreciate the size of the reabsorptive task which is carried out by the tubules. In the average healthy male, for example, 180 liters of fluid pass through the glomeruli every twenty-four hours; all but two liters are reabsorbed in the tubules. However, the role of the tubule in reducing the large quantity of glomerular filtrate is only one facet of its function. Its capacity to alter the composition of the tubular fluid by secretion is of equal importance.

Passive and Active Transport—The transport processes in tubular reabsorption are of two types—*passive* and *active*. Transport is assumed to be passive if it can be attributed to physical forces. In biological systems, such forces are due most commonly to differences in concentration or electrical potential which create gradients across membranes.

For example, when conditions are appropriate, water leaves the collecting duct because of the greater salt concentration in the surrounding medullary interstitium. Accordingly, we say the movement of water occurs because of an osmotic gradient and imply by the statement that only physical forces are operative. Therefore, the process is passive (see also page 106). Urea moves from a region where its concentration is high (tubular fluid) to one of lower concentration (peritubular blood) by diffusion; thus, its transport also is passive.

In contrast, active transport requires cellular or metabolic energy which is chemical in nature. To establish the high salt concentration in the medullary interstitium, sodium ions (with appropriate anions) are removed from a fluid in which their concentration is relatively low (as in the ascending limb) and placed in one with a substantially higher concentration. Obviously, such transport cannot proceed of its own accord any more than water can flow uphill. The required "push" is supplied by the so-called "sodium pumps" whose operations depend on chemical energy transformations. These require appropriate compounds—that is, compounds which are

capable (because of the types of atoms the contain and their arrangement) of supplyin energy for such activities and which must l provided by the cell's metabolism. Thus, tl transport of sodium is described as an acti\ process.

Tubular Reabsorption—Various substanc of metabolic importance undergo acti\

BOX 5

THE FATE OF GLUCOSE IN THE NEPHRON

The fate of glucose may be described by a simple equation involving glomerular filtration rate (GFR plasma glucose concentration (P_G), and rate of urinary glucose excretion (U_GV).

Because the concentration of glucose in glomerular fluid is the same as in plasma, it follows that tl amount of glucose which enters the nephron per unit of time, the glucose load, is determined by tl rate of glomerular filtration (GFR) and by the plasma concentration of glucose (P_G); i.e., it is tl product of the two factors GFR and P_G.

The glucose load (GFR • P_G) undergoes reabsorption either in part or completely. Establishir which of these has occurred requires estimation of glucose in urine (U_G). When this is not zero ar the rate of urine flow (V) is also known, the product (U_GV) gives the rate of urinary glucose excretior

When the urinary excretion rate (U_GV) is subtracted from the glucose load (GFR • P_G), the gluco. reabsorption rate (T_G) is obtained:

$$T_G = (GFR \cdot P_G) - U_GV$$

Indicating units:

$$T_G \text{ (mg./min.)} = \left[GFR \text{ (ml./min.)} \cdot P_G \text{ (mg./ml.)} \right] - U_GV \text{ (mg./ml.)}$$
$$T_G \text{ (mg./min.)} = (GFR \cdot P_G) \text{ (mg./min.)} - U_GV \text{ (mg./ml.)}$$

Data for an average male in health:

$$GFR = 120 \text{ ml./min.}$$
$$P_G = 1 \text{ mg./ml.}$$
$$U_G = 0; \text{ hence, } U_GV = 0$$

Substitution of these data gives:

$$T_G = (120 \text{ ml./min.} \cdot 1 \text{ mg./ml.}) - 0$$
$$T_G = 120 \text{ mg./min.}$$

Conclusions: The rate at which glucose was filtered by the glomeruli (120 mg. per minute) equaled i. rate of tubular reabsorption (120 mg. per minute); therefore, none appeared in the urine. (The reabsorr tion rate calculated from such data may be the maximum, but additional information is needed to estal lish this.)

nsport or reabsorption. However, since ucose reabsorption has been studied exten ely and is considered typical, it will be ed as a model in further discussion.

Inasmuch as glucose is freely filtered by the glomerulus, its concentration in glomerular fluid and in plasma is the same. Except for traces, glucose is not present in normal urine;

BOX 6

DETERMINATION OF RENAL PLASMA FLOW

he substance commonly used for estimation of renal plasma flow is p-aminohippurate (PAH). The moval of PAH from the blood occurs via filtration and tubular secretion. The rate of PAH filtration vends on the glomerular filtration rate (GFR) and the PAH concentration in plasma ($P_{PAH}f$), cor ted for the small amount bound to albumin. The excretion rate in urine is the product of urinary centration (U_{PAH}) and urine flow rate (V). The difference between PAH filtration rate and urinary cretion rate is PAH tubular secretion rate, expressed as follows:

$$T_{PAH} = (U_{PAH}V) - (GFR \cdot P_{PAH}f)$$

ith low concentrations (2 mg. per 100 ml.), it is assumed that PAH is completely removed from the asma in the portion of blood which perfuses the kidney's functional tissue. (Blood which perfuses er portions of the kidneys, such as the capsule and connective tissue, represents about 8 percent of total renal arterial flow. Accordingly, the PAH procedure measures an effective renal plasma w, not a true renal plasma flow.) It follows, then, that the amount of PAH removed was the entire ount present in the plasma. Furthermore, if it is assumed that all PAH removed from plasma appears the urine, the rate of PAH removal in the steady state is given by the rate of urinary excretion—i.e., 1H concentration in urine (U_{PAH}) × rate of urine flow (V). With these simplifying assumptions, ective renal plasma flow (ERPF)* may be calculated thus:

$$ERPF = \frac{Rate\ of\ urinary\ PAH\ excretion}{Plasma\ PAH\ concentration}$$

ith units indicated:

$$ERPF = \frac{U_{PAH} \cdot V\ (mg./min.)}{P_{PAH}\ (mg./ml.)} = \frac{U_{PAH}V}{P_{PAH}}\ (ml./min.)$$

ata for an average male in health:

$$U_{PAH} = 6.5\ mg./ml.$$
$$V = 1\ ml./min.$$
$$P_{PAH} = 0.01\ mg./ml.$$

bstituting these data into the equation:

$$ERPF = \frac{6.5\ (mg./ml.) \cdot 1\ (ml./min.)}{0.01\ (mg./ml.)} = \frac{6.5\ (mg./min.)}{0.01\ (mg./ml.)} = 650\ ml./min.$$

---

he equation for calculation of ERPF is based on the Fick principle with modifications appropriate to the present case.

therefore, it must be reabsorbed in the tubules. Because the tubular concentration of glucose becomes virtually zero, its transport occurs against a steep concentration gradient and depends on an active transport mechanism of great importance for health.

In health, urine remains free of glucose even when the amount in plasma increases owing, for example, to an intake of food. Under normal conditions, the clearance of glucose is zero; all glucose that is filtered becomes reabsorbed. Accordingly, the rate of tubular reabsorption is not constant but must keep pace with the plasma level. Above a critical plasma level, however, glucose does appear in the urine, and the amount increases in proportion to any increase in the plasma. In effect, the absorption rate has a maximum, and when this is reached, additional glucose is not reabsorbed but remains in the tubules to be excreted with the urine.

Other substances, including amino acids, phosphate, sulfate, and urate, are actively reabsorbed by the tubules in a similar way. Active reabsorptive processes (except those for water and the monovalent ions) are confined to the proximal convoluted tubule.

Tubular Secretion—A great number of substances are transported from the peritubular capillaries to the tubular lumen. Tubular secretion (also referred to as "tubular excretion") occurs with ionic organic compounds such as sulfonic acids, carboxylic acids, amines, some iodinated compounds used in radiography, glucuronides, and various antibiotics, of which penicillin is an important example. It is also the means by which the inorganic ions potassium, hydrogen, and ammonium enter the urine. (The secretion of hydrogen ions is discussed in the next section.)

Tubular secretion is the major route for elimination of toxic metabolic products and foreign substances, including drugs. Although a few drugs are filtered in the glomerul most are not, because they are bound t plasma proteins. Removal of the compound from plasma is left to the tubular cells, which may be so efficient that virtually all of the bound material is removed in a single circulation through the kidney. This is the wa penicillin is eliminated.

Tubular secretion of organic ions appea to depend on two separate transport mecha nisms—one for the anions and another for th cations. Neither system is highly specific sinc each transports a wide variety of organic compounds with the appropriate electric charge. Competition for transport has bee demonstrated with many compounds an has important consequences in therapy.

The avidity of the tubular secretory system for certain organic anions and efficient re moval of these from peritubular blood ar properties utilized to measure renal plasm flow. From such data, renal blood flow ca be calculated.

The Secretion of Hydrogen Ions and th Regeneration of Bicarbonate—The kidney remarkable capacity for acidification (and therefore, their importance in maintainin acid-base balance) is particularly evident du ing severe acidosis, when the hydrogen-io concentration may be 1,000 times greater i urine than in plasma. Such a large differenc is possible because of an ion-exchange mecha nism which operates in the proximal and dis tal tubules and in the collecting duct. Briefly hydrogen ions are exchanged for sodiu ions; that is, the hydrogen ions are trans ported across luminal cell borders into tubu lar and collecting duct fluid while sodiu ions move in the opposite direction an finally enter the bloodstream. Along wit the movement of these ions, bicarbonate i regenerated and also enters the bloodstream.

The direct source of the hydrogen ions secreted is uncertain. It may be carbonic acid (H_2CO_3), which is produced by the carbonic-anhydrase-catalyzed hydration of CO_2—i.e., $H_2O + CO_2 \rightleftharpoons H_2CO_3$. Other more complex reactions have been postulated. A schematic representation of the ion exchange and bicarbonate regeneration is in Figure 55.

Secreted hydrogen ions react with the tubular fluid's bicarbonate, phosphate, or ammonia. Obviously, these or similar reactions are essential to dispose of hydrogen ions and prevent rapid attainment of a limiting *p*H, about 4.5 in man, and resulting cessation of

hydrogen-ion secretion. The major buffers in blood (and, consequently, in glomerular filtrate and in tubular fluid) are bicarbonate and phosphate, with the former greatly predominating in amount. Accordingly, most of the hydrogen ions secreted react with bicarbonate. The carbonic acid so formed decomposes spontaneously and/or catalytically, when carbonic anhydrase is present, to CO_2 and water. Since CO_2 is freely diffusible, it enters the tubular cells and adds to the pool which is the source of CO_2 for carbonic-anhydrase-catalyzed synthesis of carbonic acid.

The renal ion-exchange mechanism of Figure 55 has been modified in Figure 56 to show specifically the role of sodium bicarbonate as a hydrogen-ion acceptor. According to the scheme, the bicarbonate of blood, which entered the nephron via glomerular filtrate and was decomposed by tubular-se-

Figure 55. Schematic representation of renal ion exchange and bicarbonate regeneration. In tubular cells, hydration of CO_2, catalyzed by carbonic anhydrase (CA), yields carbonic acid (H_2CO_3), and dissociation of this produces the hydrogen ion, which is secreted into tubular fluid in exchange for a sodium ion. The thick curved arrows represent coupled active transport reactions without identification of the second component. Other transport, including diffusion, is shown by dashes. For each hydrogen ion secreted into the tubule, one bicarbonate ion is returned to the blood.

Figure 56. The renal ion-exchange mechanism with bicarbonate as the hydrogen-ion acceptor in tubular fluid. The CO_2 produced by decomposition of the bicarbonate may diffuse from tubular fluid and enter the CO_2 pool in the tubular cells.

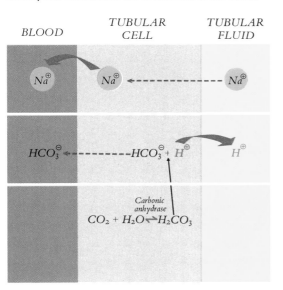

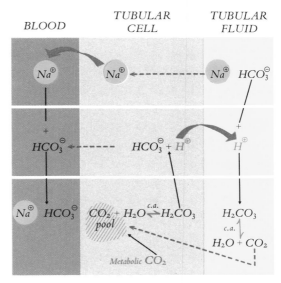

creted hydrogen ions, is regenerated in tubular cells and makes its way back into the bloodstream.

Reaction with phosphate and ammonia, as with bicarbonate, fits the renal scheme (Figure 55). The three reactions differ in the substance which acts as acceptor of the secreted hydrogen ions. Thus, disodium phosphate is converted to monosodium phosphate (Figure 57), and ammonia becomes ammonium ion (Figure 58), but the renal ion exchange and bicarbonate regeneration scheme remain unchanged.

The reaction with phosphate occurs mostly in the distal tubule and in the collecting duct. This reaction and those with buffers present in small amounts (hence of lesser importance) —but not with bicarbonate and ammonia— yield acidic compounds which are titratable. Accordingly, the amount of base required to bring urine to its initial pH of 7.4 (the pH of glomerular filtrate) is called its *titratable acidity*. This amount, however, represents only a fraction of the total secreted hydrogen ions.

Ammonia is secreted in the proximal and distal tubules and in the collecting duct. It diffuses easily through cell membranes because of its solubility in lipids, in contrast to ammonium ion, which remains in tubular fluid and is eliminated via urine.

Filtration, Tubular Reabsorption, and Secretion—Some substances—notably potassium but probably also phosphate and uric acid—enter the nephron in the glomerular filtrate, undergo reabsorption in the proximal tubule, and appear in the urine largely as a result of secretion in the distal tubule. This is the sequence of events in health. In disease, the site of damage may alter the relative importance of the tubular functions. Thus, damage in the proximal segment may result in failure of reabsorption and cause excessive urinary loss. If the disease is located in the distal tubule, secretion may be impaired enough to bring about abnormal retention.

Figure 57. The renal ion-exchange mechanism with dibasic phosphate as the hydrogen acceptor.

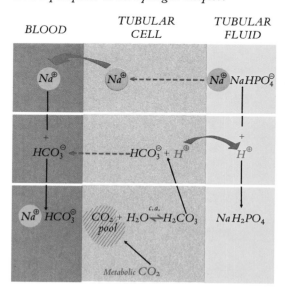

Figure 58. The renal ion-exchange mechanism with ammonia as the hydrogen acceptor.

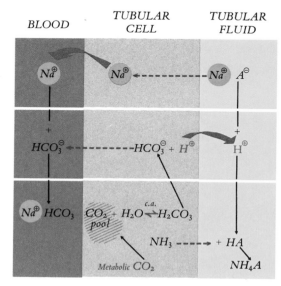

CONCENTRATING AND DILUTING MECHANISM

By the time vertebrates had completed their migration from fresh water to land, the kidney's mechanism for maintaining body fluids at constant volume had been drastically changed. In the former aquatic environment, the problem was solved by a process of water excretion. On land the opposite was necessary: Water had to be conserved. Consequently, a mechanism to produce urine considerably more concentrated than the body fluids from which it originated finally evolved and became the distinguishing feature of avian and mammalian renal function.

Iso-osmotic Reabsorption—The osmolality of glomerular fluid and plasma is virtually identical because the glomerular capillaries are freely permeable to nearly all components of plasma except its proteins. (The contribution made by proteins to the glomerular fluid's colligative properties is relatively slight in comparison with that made by particles present in much greater numbers, such as the electrolytes and other small molecules. For a discussion of colligative properties, see Box 7.)

BOX 7

COLLIGATIVE PROPERTIES OF SOLUTIONS

Colligative properties of solutions have the common characteristic of dependence only on the relative number of solute and solvent particles and hence, ideally, are not influenced by the nature of the solute. Examples are osmotic pressure and freezing-point depression. The latter is commonly used to define solutions. Thus, the freezing point of a solution consisting of one gram-molecular weight of any undissociated substance dissolved in 1,000 Gm. of water will be $-1.86°C$. This is an osmolal solution because it contains 1 osmol of solute particles in 1,000 Gm. of water (i.e., the number of particles required to lower the freezing point of water by $1.86°C$.). Osmolality is an expression of concentration in terms of 1,000 Gm. of water. Accordingly, neither temperature nor the space taken up by the solids present in the solution has any bearing on the osmolality figure, and a direct comparison can be made of various body fluids with different water—or solids—content.

On the other hand, such a comparison is not possible when concentration is expressed in terms of 1 liter of solution—i.e., osmolarity. The amount of water in 1 liter of solution is a function both of its temperature and the space occupied by the solids in solution. Inasmuch as colligative properties are determined only by the ratio of solute to solvent particles, the osmolarity of various body fluids is not directly comparable.

In the absence of dissociation, each molecule of solute behaves as a single particle; therefore, 1 osmol is one gram-molecular weight. Therefore—and because difference in molecular size has no effect on colligative properties—one gram-molecular weight of albumin (mol. wt. 70,000) affects the freezing point of water to the same degree as one gram-molecular weight of urea (mol. wt. 60). If dissociation occurs—as with sodium chloride, for example—and two ions are formed, each molecule has the effect of two particles. In this case, then, 1 osmol is one-half of the molecular weight.

To avoid decimals in discussing physiological solutions, the units milliosmol and microosmol are used to represent one-thousandth and one-millionth osmols respectively. Thus, in health, the osmotic concentrations of plasma and extracellular fluid are nearly 300 milliosmolal (mOsm).

Figure 59. *The principal parts of a juxtamedullary nephron and related structures appear in the diagram on the left. Their functions, which will be described in stepwise fashion, are represented on the right. Portions of the nephron are delineated by colors, with the gradation of color in each section indicating change in composition or in concentration of the fluid present. Thus, the gradation of color in the medullary interstitium represents the change in osmolality indicated by numbers.*

Step 1. Blood reaches the glomerulus via the afferent arteriole and leaves via the efferent arteriole. The filtrate formed flows from Bowman's capsule into the proximal tubule, where reabsorption of solutes and water occurs. The copious blood supply of the peritubular capillaries returns these substances into the general circulation.

Step 2. The descending limb is permeable to water and is surrounded by an interstitium in which the salt concentration increases from cortex to papilla. As the fluid within the limb flows downward, it is exposed to osmotic pressure created by this salt gradient, and water is lost by osmosis (as indicated by the wavy lines). (The change in salt concentration of the fluid is represented by transition of color from blue to green.)

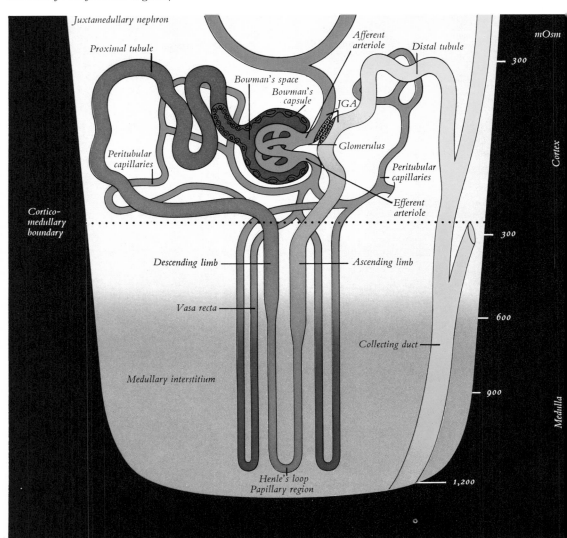

Step 3. When the loop's turn brings the fluid into the ascending limb, the flow becomes countercurrent. Pumps transfer salt (i.e., sodium ions) out of the ascending limb (which is impermeable to water) into the interstitium. The pumps at any given level transport sodium ions against a slight gradient (represented by the inclined lines). The decrease in the tubular fluid's solute concentration is indicated by gradation of color from green to yellow-green.

Step 4. The fluid that enters the distal tubule is relatively hypotonic (represented by the yellow-green color). By the time it leaves, however, it has been restored to isotonicity (shown in yellow). The distal tubule is the site of active sodium transport and passive loss of water together with excretion of hydrogen and potassium ions.

Step 5. The fluid in the collecting duct is subjected to the osmotic forces in the medullary interstitium. However, the duct's permeability is under hormonal control, and loss of water by osmosis (wavy lines) is governed by the body's total requirements. The increase in concentration of the collecting duct fluid is shown by the shading of the color.

Step 6. In the medulla, blood is supplied by the vasa recta. The loop arrangement of vessels permits countercurrent flow (indicated by the curved arrows). The direction of flow together with its slow rate allows substances to pass into these vessels as they penetrate the medulla (deepening red color) and out of them on the outward journey (fading of color).

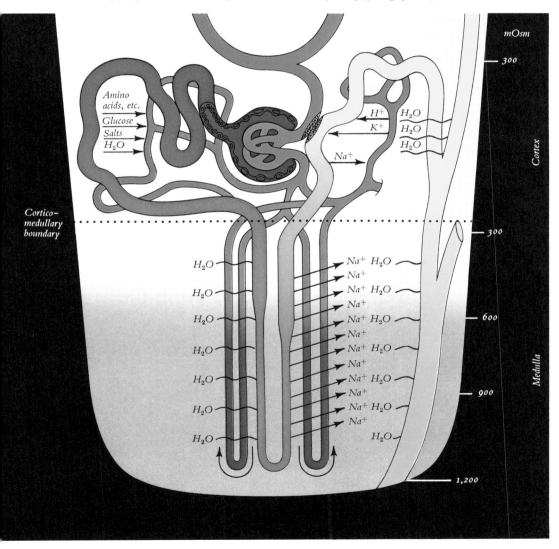

The glomerular filtrate flows from Bowman's capsule into the extensively convoluted proximal tubule, where almost all of its glucose, amino acids, and other metabolites and much of its sodium chloride are reabsorbed (Figure 59, Step 1). The membranes on the luminal cells of the proximal tubule are water permeable; hence, the active transport processes are accompanied by a passive movement of water. In this way, nearly 80 percent of the water in the glomerular filtrate is reabsorbed within the proximal segment without change in osmolality of the fluid that remains. Accordingly, the process may be described as *iso-osmotic reabsorption*. Data on luminal fluid obtained by micropuncture indicate that the events described occur during water deprivation and hydration.

Structure and Relationship of Capillaries and Tubules

The rapid and extensive exchange between tubules and the vascular network in the cortex is facilitated by the structure of the peritubular capillaries and the tubular cells. The capillary wall is thin and contains numerous round fenestrations resembling those in the glomerulus; each is apparently covered by a "diaphragm" with a central knob. Furthermore, since capillaries and tubules are in close proximity, reabsorbed substances traverse a very short distance before reaching the capillary stream (Figure 60).

The cells of the proximal tubule have fine projections, the brush border, on the luminal surface (Figures 61 and 62a). Such projections greatly increase the area that is in contact with tubular fluid and thereby promote reabsorption by either active or passive means. Between the projections, the surface membrane forms invaginations (Figure 61) which appear to develop into vacuoles; possibly these are the mechanism for taking in molecules too large to pass through luminal membranes.

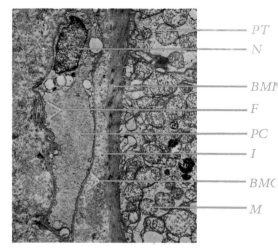

Figure 60. The peritubular capillary (PC) lies close to the proximal tubule (PT). The wall of the capillary is thin and contains numerous fenestrations (F); these are present here only in cross section and hence resemble a string of approximately oval beads. Other structures of the capillary are the endothelial cell nucleus (N) and the basement membrane (BMC). The proximal tubule cell contains numerous mitochondria (M) and is enveloped by a prominent basement membrane (BMP). The interstitium (I) contains a collagen-like material (electron micrograph, 8,200×).

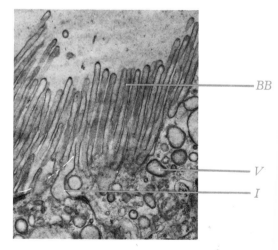

Figure 61. Portion of proximal tubule cell showing brush border (BB) with invaginations (I) and vacuoles (V) (electron micrograph, 28,375×).

The numerous mitochondria (Figure 62a) indicate the high level of oxidative enzyme activity needed to supply the energy for active transport.

The Medulla—When the fluid leaves the proximal convoluted tubule and enters the descending limb of Henle's loop, it passes from the cortical to the medullary portion of the kidney and enters the region where concentration and dilution of urine take place. The essential structures for this phase of renal function are Henle's loop (with its thick descending and ascending limbs, thin descending and ascending segments, and the hairpin turn), the medullary interstitium, the collecting duct, and the concomitant vasculature.

Significance of Henle's Loop—For many years it has been known that Henle's loop is present in the kidneys of only those animals which produce a concentrated urine—i.e., birds and mammals. Furthermore, there is a relationship between length of loop and degree of concentrating ability. For example, beavers have a predominance of relatively short-loop nephrons and a correspondingly limited concentrating ability. In contrast, some desert rodents that have unusually long loops produce urine with an osmolality as much as nine times greater than that of plasma. Man and dog are intermediate, with a mixture of nephrons containing short and long loops.

Length of Henle's Loop—In man, the length of Henle's loop, especially that of the thin segment, is related to the location of the renal corpuscle of its origin (Figure 63). When it lies close to the corticomedullary boundary (and hence is part of a *juxtamedullary nephron*), the loop is characteristically long and penetrates deeply into the medulla. In some in-stances it may reach the papilla. In contrast, the *cortical nephron* has a considerably shorter loop (Figure 63), since its renal corpuscle is some distance removed from the cortical boundary. In the case of cortical nephrons that originate in the outer portion of the cortex, the thin segment may be absent, and the loop may not reach the medulla.

The Configuration of Henle's Loop—The arrangement of Henle's loop in the form of a hairpin is the anatomic feature essential to its function of establishing and maintaining a gradient of salt concentration in the medullary interstitium which, in turn, is directly responsible for concentrating the urine. Furthermore, the two limbs of the loop are physiologically unlike and play dissimilar roles. The descending portion is freely permeable to water and readily loses water by osmosis to the interstitium. In contrast, the ascending limb is watertight and contains "pumps" to transport sodium ions from tubular fluid to interstitium; in this way, its osmotic gradient is maintained.

The Descending Limb—The descending limb of Henle's loop consists of a thick portion, which is the terminal part of the proximal tubule, and a thin segment. The transition between these structures is fairly abrupt. It consists of a change in type of epithelium from columnar to flat squamous and a considerable decrease in tube diameter (Figure 62b). The cells of the thin segment contain only a few mitochondria (as compared with proximal tubule cells) and almost no brush border. This suggests that neither active transport nor reabsorption is an important function in the thin segment.

As the descending limb penetrates into the medulla, it is subjected to a spectrum of osmotic forces ranging from that of plasma

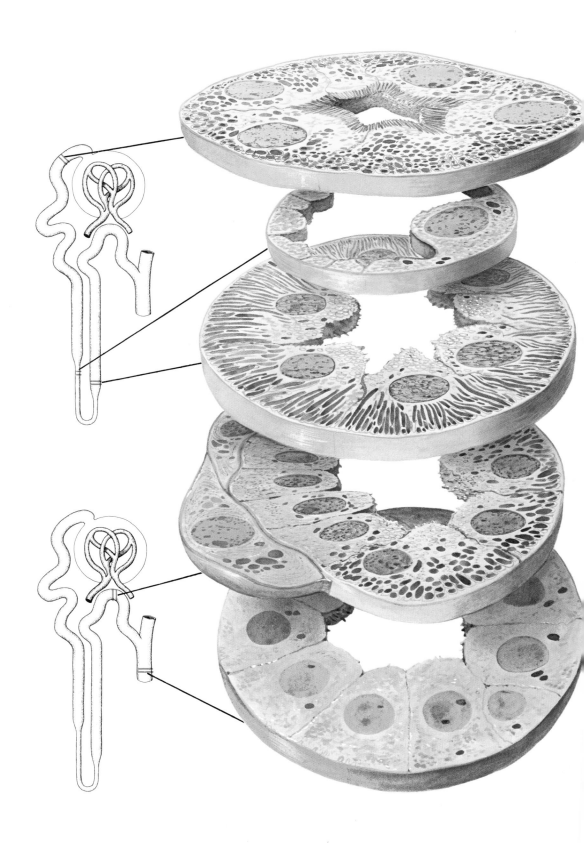

Figure 62. Essential cellular features in different parts of the kidney tubules.

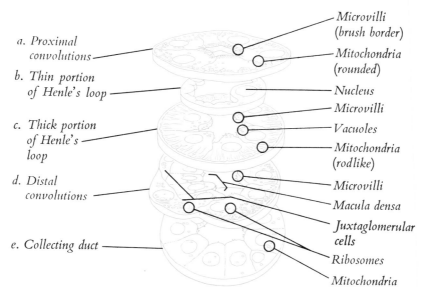

a. Proximal convolutions

b. Thin portion of Henle's loop

c. Thick portion of Henle's loop

d. Distal convolutions

e. Collecting duct

Microvilli (brush border)

Mitochondria (rounded)

Nucleus

Microvilli

Vacuoles

Mitochondria (rodlike)

Microvilli

Macula densa

Juxtaglomerular cells

Ribosomes

Mitochondria

(about 300 mOsm) at the corticomedullary boundary to as much as 1,200 mOsm in the papillary region (Figure 59, Step 2).

Since forces produced by this gradient remove water from the fluid as it flows down the descending limb, its solute concentration rises and approximately equals that of the interstitium at corresponding levels. In this way, tubular fluid is made progressively more concentrated by *osmosis*, from cortex to papilla, and may reach 1,200 mOsm by the time it makes the turn in the loop.

The Ascending Limb—The ascending limb passes through the medullary interstitium in a direction opposite to that taken by the descending limb (Figure 59, Step 3). Furthermore, these limbs lie close together, and any space between them is bridged by interstitial material; therefore, both are in essentially identical osmotic environments.

When the greatly concentrated fluid makes the turn and enters the ascending limb, it begins to flow *countercurrent*, literally retracing its steps. As the fluid flows toward the cortex, pumps transfer sodium ions out of the tubule into the medullary interstitium.

At any level, the concentration of solute in the interstitium is only slightly greater than that in the tubular fluid. This difference in corresponding levels is maintained from the papillary to the cortical zones of the medulla. Accordingly, the most concentrated *tubular fluid* is the source of sodium ions for that portion of the *interstitium* correspondingly highest in solute. As the fluid moves up the ascending limb, it becomes progressively less concentrated and serves as a source of sodium ions for a progressively less concentrated interstitium. Thus, the countercurrent arrangement permits the sodium pumps to work against only a small gradient. However,

Figure 63. In the mammalian kidney, the length of Henle's loop is related to the position of its renal corpuscle in the cortex.

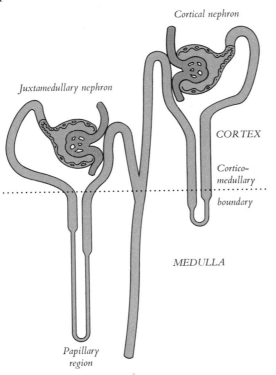

ascending limb gradually changes into the distal convoluted tubule (Figure 62d). Also, their number diminishes, so that, at the terminal portions of the convoluted tubule, only a few are present in each cell. The luminal surface of cells both in the thick portion and in the distal convoluted tubule is provided with many microvilli. These projections, however, are not as fine as those in the proximal tubule, nor are they as numerous (Figures 62a and 62c). In the apical region of each cell there is an abundance of small vesicles (Figure 62c). Their function is uncertain, but they resemble the vacuoles in the acid-producing parietal cells of the gastric mucosa. Accordingly, it has been suggested that they are involved in the mechanism for acidification of urine.

Ribosomes are present in abundance in the cells of the distal convoluted tubule. Most are free, but some may be attached to ribbon-like membranes to form the typical endoplasmic reticulum.

The Distal Tubule—When the fluid in the ascending limb reaches the corticomedullary boundary and enters the distal convoluted tubule, it is relatively hypotonic (i.e., 200 to 230 mOsm). Active sodium transport continues here and may be accompanied by passive loss of water. In addition, excretion of potassium and hydrogen ions occurs in the distal tubule (Figure 59, Step 4).

Two groups of specialized cells located in this region play important roles in hormonal control of kidney function and are discussed below. When the distal convoluted tubule reaches the renal corpuscle of its origin, it makes contact with the afferent arteriole just before this vessel enters Bowman's capsule. The tubular cells along the line of contact are characteristically narrow with prominent nuclei (Figure 62d). These cells are the *macula densa;* together with those on the adjacent

since the pumping continues along the entire length of the ascending limb, the pumping step is repeated over and over, and its small effect is multiplied many times—hence, the term *countercurrent multiplier system.* In this way, a salt concentration gradient is formed from papilla to cortex with a range far greater than could be produced by any single-step pumping mechanism known in a biological system.

The thick portion of the ascending limb resembles the thick descending limb. It is approximately the same diameter, and its cuboidal cells contain a large number of mitochondria, although these are characteristically rod-shaped (Figure 62c). The rod-shaped mitochondria become more ovoid as the wall of the afferent arteriole (Figure 62d), they make up the *juxtaglomerular apparatus* (JGA) (Figure 59).

Hormonal Control—The various components and their relationships in the hormonal con-trol of kidney function, to which reference is made in the following discussion, appear in Figure 64. Changes in the sodium con-centration of the tubular fluid, as well as in the rate or volume of flow itself, are sensed by the cells of the *macula densa*, which cause

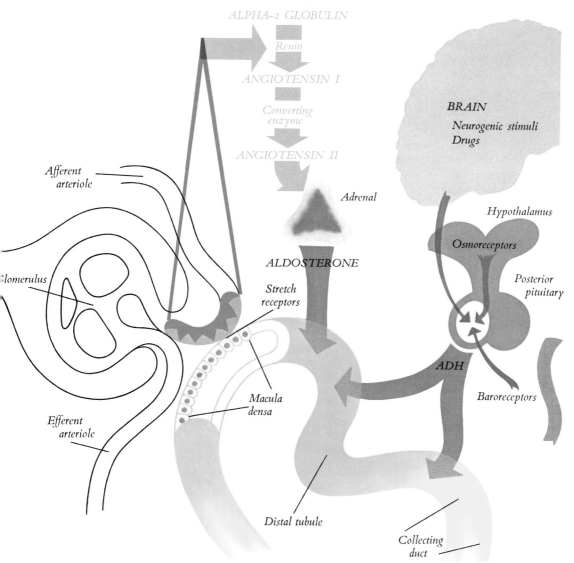

Figure 64. Schematic representation of hormonal control of kidney function. The products formed in enzymatic reactions and the enzymes are shown in blue. Hormones are shown in magenta, with arrows leading from their point of origin to the site of action. The stimuli which reach the posterior pituitary are represented by gray arrows.

the adjacent *stretch receptors* in the wall of the arteriole to release appropriate amounts of the enzyme *renin*. In the blood, renin splits an *alpha-2 globulin*, one of the plasma proteins, into a ten-peptide structure, *angiotensin I*, which loses two amino acids via a *converting enzyme* to become the eight-peptide vasopressor substance *angiotension II*. This is the material that reaches the adrenal cortex and triggers the release of the hormone *aldosterone*. The rate of sodium reabsorption in the *distal tubule* is under direct control of this hormone. By adjustment of renin release to control aldosterone secretion, the amount of sodium that will appear in urine is determined in the distal tubule in response to the body's total requirements.

In the hypothalamic area of the brain, cells sensitive to osmotic pressure (*osmoreceptors*) detect changes in the solute concentration of the plasma bathing them. The neurogenic signals they send to the *posterior pituitary* cause release of an eight-membered chain of amino acids—*vasopressin*, or *antidiuretic hormone* (ADH). ADH release can also be triggered by *neurogenic stimuli*, such as shock, pain, and trauma; by certain *drugs*, such as morphine, ether, and nicotine; and by a fall in vascular volume, as in hemorrhage, noted by *baroreceptors*. The antidiuretic hormone controls the rate of water reabsorption in both the *distal tubule* and the *collecting duct*. It acts by altering the permeability of those ducts; more or less water is allowed to escape into the interstitium and to be conserved in response to the body's total needs.

The Collecting Ducts—When the distal tubule fluid, now restored to isotonicity, again crosses the corticomedullary boundary, it enters the system of collecting ducts (Figure 59, Step 5). These structures are in the medulla; hence, the fluid they carry is exposed to the spectrum of osmotic forces from cortex to papilla. Here, as in the distal tubule, permeability is under control of the antidiuretic hormone. For this reason, the amount of water lost by osmosis to the interstitium—and, thus, the degree of urine concentration—depends on the body's total water requirements. In the extreme situation, the solute concentration may approach 1,200 mOsm, the osmolality of the medulla in the papillary region.

The collecting duct consists of simple epithelium throughout its length (Figure 62e). However, the cell type changes gradually from cuboidal in the cortex to columnar in the papillary zone, where groups of collecting ducts are joined to form the large duct of Bellini. All collecting duct cells contain short, coarse microvilli on the luminal surface, and vesicles are present in the cell's apex. Neither mitochondria nor ribosomes are abundant, although some cells have more than others. So far, the site of action of the antidiuretic hormone on collecting duct cells has not been identified.

The Vasa Recta—The circulation of blood in the medullary interstitium, without destruction of its osmotic gradient, is carried out by the vasa recta (Figure 59, Step 6). The medulla's vascular system has two unique features which permit it to function in the required way: The blood flow is slower here than it is in vessels elsewhere, and the vessels themselves do not pass through the medulla in one direction but, instead, are arranged in loop form so that each enters and leaves in approximately the same area.

The slow blood flow in the vasa recta allows time for equilibration during passage into the medulla and out of it. Thus, when blood enters the medulla, it is about 300 nOsm but may become as much as 1,200 nOsm by the time it reaches the papillary zone and changes its direction of flow. On the outward journey, equilibration continues, but now the solute concentration is diminished. The blood is slightly hypo-osmolal when it reaches the region of the corticomedullary boundary, as might be expected, since it is carrying water out of the medullary interstitium.

The loop arrangement of the vasa recta allows for countercurrent flow and is the device (together with the slow rate of flow) by which the concentration changes the blood undergoes while moving in one direction are almost completely undone during its flow in the opposite direction. (Accordingly, this is called the *countercurrent exchange system*.) The small difference is all-important, because it is sufficient to prevent accumulation of water in the medulla without destroying its osmotic gradient.

GENERAL REFERENCES

Becker, E. L. (Editor): Structural Basis of Renal Disease. New York: Hoeber Medical Division, Harper & Row, Publishers, 1968.

Berliner, R. W., Levinsky, N. G., Davidson, D. G., and Eden, M.: Dilution and Concentration of the Urine and the Action of Antidiuretic Hormone, Am. J. Med., 24:730, 1958.

Black, D. A. K.: Essentials of Fluid Balance, Ed. 2. Oxford: Blackwell Scientific Publications, 1960.

Elkinton, J. R., and Danowski, T. S.: The Body Fluids. Baltimore: The Williams & Wilkins Company, 1955.

Giebisch, G., and Windhager, E. E.: Renal Tubular Transfer of Sodium, Chloride and Potassium, Am. J. Med., 36:643, 1964.

Gottschalk, C. W.: Renal Tubular Function: Lessons from Micropuncture, Harvey Lect., 58:99, 1963.

Kessler, R. H.: Physiologic Basis of Fluid and Electrolyte Therapy, Mod. Treat., 5:617, 1968.

Pitts, R. F.: Physiology of the Kidney and Body Fluids, Ed. 2. Chicago: Year Book Medical Publishers, Inc., 1968.

Pitts, R. F.: The Physiological Basis of Diuretic Therapy. Springfield: Charles C Thomas, Publisher, 1959.

Smith, H. W.: Principles of Renal Physiology. New York: Oxford University Press, 1956.

Wirz, H., Hangitay, B., and Kuhn, W.: Lokalisation des Konzentrierungsprozesses in der Niere durch direkte Kryoskopie, Helvet. physiol. et pharmacol. acta, 9:196, 1951.

Filius. Mechelebria. Id eft, ferculum, quod fit ex carnibus, uzo, & lacte, & fpeciebus calidis. Eft ci-
Ma. bus temperatus, bonus temperatis complexionibus. Temperantia uero fua eft in eo,
quod caliditas conuertitur ex frigiditate rizon, & obtemperatur ficcitas rizon,
æquata lactis humiditati. Et eft de cibis quiefcentium, & exercitantium
moderate, & maxime temporibus temperatis. Qui cibus nec
conftrictiuus, nec laxatiuus exiftens, purificat in-
tellectum, & delectabilia fomnia efficit.

Filius. Pumata, & Kibelia. Eliguntur hæc duo fercula habentibus complexiones cholericas,
Alb. & habentibus ftomachum debilem, & habentibus hepar calidum, uel inflam-
matum, & habentibus diuturnum fluxum cholericum: & communi-
cantur patientibus afperitatem pectoris & pulmonis: & co-
licis, habentibus complexiones frigidas. Et funt
nociua neruis. Sunt etiam offendentes fper-
ma & coitum, minuentes appetitum.

Ma. Rapata, & Cumabitia. Eliguntur huiufmodi fercula caulium, habentibus complexiones frigidas. Gumebet eft maneries caulis, cuius flos magnus & grofsus, ficut unum uas
magnum. Et odiuntur, quia flegma generant, faciunt uentofitates, & dolores fortes. Et
bona funt ad prouocandam urinam, & maxime quando præparantur oua caulium ipforum tantum: & quando elixantur cum aqua & fale huiufmodi caules, funt nocui ftomacho. Rapata uero calida eft & humida, addens in coitu, quia uentofitatum eft generatiua:
quæ cum bene digeritur, nutrit nutrimento multo & bono.

Filius. Dififcera. Eft ferculum acetofum, factum de carnibus, & fucco acetofo, & muri. Eliguntur
Ma. Dififcera habentibus humidum ftomachum, & plenum flegmate. Verumtamen eft noci-
uum melancholiæ, & habentibus complexiones frigidas & ficcas, & macilentis. Et hic cibus
conficif ex Afkipitio muri, feu uini: & generaliter uini eft confectio, facta ex farina grofsa (quæ
nominatur polina) fale, origano, & aqua: quæ conferuatur ad ufum. Hic cibus habet multas
diuerfas operationes: eo quod in eo funt plures & diuerfi fapores, uidelicet, dulcedo, acetofi-
tas, et falfedo: et fecundū hanc rationē complexio eius dicif a complexione uincētis.

Ra. Rizon, et Milium præparatum cum lacte. Eligitur hic cibus factus ex Rizon, uel ex Milio
cum lacte, eo quod fac humectat ficcitatem ipforum: & fit propterea cibus temperatus in
humiditate & ficcitate, inclinans ad frigiditatem: quæ nutrit corpus multum: & quando comeditur cum zuccaro, uel melle, uelocius digeritur. Verumtamen eft cibus inconueniens habentibus opilationem renum & hepatis, & illis in quorum renibus generatur lapis. Verum
Milium, & Panicium, & Rizon funt frigidiora, licet fint æqualia in ficcitate.
Quidam tamen dixerunt, quod Rizon calefacit calefactos.

Iudæ- Magumimæ. Sunt carnes præparatæ cum aceto in uafe fictili, cuius orificium fit obtura-
us. tum cum cæra, feu pafta. De proprietate huius ferculi, eft incidere flegma cum falfedine
& acetofitate, quæ funt in eo: & eft humorum fubtiliatiuum, & nutrit abundanter quando digeritur. Verum replet caput acutis uaporibus, & obeft cerebro & neruis. Eft
malum habentibus ftomachos debiles. Et poft hunc cibum diliguntur
a quibufdam Melones comech: quod eft de rebus ma-
gis offendentibus digeftionem ipfius.

Io. Maskinbe. Id eft, carnes afsæ in loco quem ignis inflammauit. Aduerfantur conuale-
fcentibus, & utentibus quiete, & ftatu, & ftomachum habentibus debilem: maxime quando comeditur cum fubtilibus cibis, uel poft comeftionem
ipfius, afsumatur cibus ftipticus: eo quod fumefcit cibus ifte in ftomacho ipforum & corrumpi-
tur. Attamen bonus eft exercitan-
tibus fortiter, & illis, quorum corpus eft calidum, & pori aperti.

Apta huc q̃
fupra fol. 21.
Canone. 24.

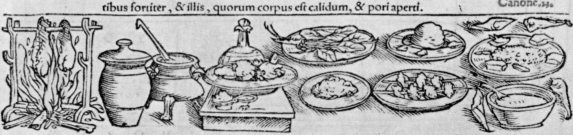

Maskinbe.   Magu-   Rizon &   Dififcera.   Rapata, &   Pumata, & Kibelia.   Mechelebria.
       mimæ.   Miliū cum lacte.   Cumabitia.

7

Management in Renal Insufficiency

*your physician does not think it wise for you
sleep, to take wine or such and such meat,
not be troubled, I will find you another who
'll not be of his opinion; the diversity of
edical arguments and opinions includes every
riety of form.*

— *Michel de Montaigne (1533–1592)*

OBJECTIVES

Three methods useful in the management of renal insufficiency, whether it is due to pyelonephritis or to any other cause, are *dietary control*, *dialysis*, and *transplantation*. The procedure or combination of procedures likely to be of value depends largely on the degree of normal renal function that remains. For example, a dietary regimen along with suitable control of water, electrolytes, and acid-base balance may be adequate until the glomerular filtration rate diminishes to about 3 ml. per minute. With further deterioration, diet alone is ineffective and must be supplemented with some method of dialysis or transplantation. In addition, judicious application of drug therapy may be beneficial at some time during the course of chronic renal failure.

The goals to be achieved with proper management of irreversible renal disease include (1) adjustment of metabolic and dietary load to fit the patient's renal capacity, (2) control of electrolyte balance and fluid volume, (3) improvement of reversible components of

of discussion on the useful or harmful effects of various foods, including those of importance to the kidneys.

Tacuini sanitatis. Strassburg, 1531. (Courtesy of the Lilly Library, Indiana University, Bloomington, Indiana) renal function, and (4) support of failing organ systems.

ALTERED PHYSIOLOGY

The severely diseased kidney has considerable difficulty in excreting the final products of protein metabolism because renal functions are greatly diminished or eliminated by destruction of the pertinent structures.[1]

The diseased kidney's glomerular filtration rate may be markedly reduced. When it falls below 25 percent of normal, there is a rise in the blood levels of nitrogenous compounds, especially urea and creatinine. With a urea level of about 150 mg. per 100 ml. of blood, various gastro-intestinal symptoms of uremia appear, including nausea, vomiting, loss of appetite, diarrhea, and melena. However, when uremia develops quickly, these signs and symptoms may occur at a lower concentration of blood urea.

The diminished filtration rate is also responsible for retention of various inorganic anions, such as the hydrogen-ion acceptors sulfate and phosphate. Furthermore, bicarbonate stores may become severely depleted because of limited bicarbonate replacement by the damaged kidneys.

Another quantitatively important acid acceptor may also be in short supply or entirely lacking. Damage to the distal convoluted tubule may adversely affect the sites of ammonia synthesis and produce a corresponding decrease in availability of ammonia (NH_3). In this way, the usual route of excretion of a substantial portion of hydrogen ions as ammonium (NH_4^+) may be severely curtailed.

The ability of tubular cells to excrete hydrogen ions is limited in the diseased kidney. Thus, since the normal exchange of hydrogen ions for sodium ions is greatly diminished, hydrogen ions are retained and sodium ions are excreted in the urine. (For a discussion of kidney functions, see Chapter 6.)

Briefly, then, the low rate of glomerular filtration in the severely diseased kidney results in nitrogen retention and may be accompanied by symptoms of uremia. There is also retention of important acid acceptors and limited replacement of bicarbonate. Damage elsewhere in the nephron affects ammonia synthesis and further reduces the means available for removal of hydrogen ions via urine. In addition, hydrogen ions are retained and sodium ions are excreted. For these reasons, nitrogen retention and acidosis in varying degrees occur in renal insufficiency and are prime factors to be dealt with if the therapeutic regimen is to prove successful.

DIET

By restriction of the daily intake of protein,[2,3] the amount of its end products which the diseased kidneys must excrete is correspondingly reduced. The extent of protein restriction needed may be judged by the patient's residual kidney function.

For the patient with urea nitrogen in excess of 50 mg. per 100 ml. of blood but with no symptoms of uremia and without marked signs of renal insufficiency, a diet containing approximately 50 Gm. of protein per day has proved acceptable. The total caloric intake should be adequate, with needed calories obtained from nonprotein foods, such as vegetable oils, pastries made with wheat starch flour, candies, carbonated beverages, jellies, sugar, honey, and fruit ices. With the anorexic patient, however, it may be impossible to maintain caloric balance.

Diets very low in protein (i.e., about 20 Gm. per day) are required for the patient with blood urea nitrogen levels higher than 100 mg. and/or a glomerular filtration rate (creatinine clearance) of less than 5 ml. per minute. Although strict control of diet may be difficult, it is generally a very rewarding therapeutic undertaking in such patients.

The protein intake in the very-low-protein diet must be sufficient to maintain nitrogen balance, and the protein used must be of high biological value so that it supplies all essential amino acids, with the possible exception of methionine. Oral supplements of methionine and vitamins are recommended.

The caloric content of very-low-protein diets should be high enough—approximately 2,000 calories. The additional calories are obtained from fats and carbohydrate foods that are essentially protein-free. It is necessary to supply sufficient amounts of fats and carbohydrates to maintain nitrogen balance on the low-protein diet and thereby prevent breakdown of endogenous protein with wasting of muscles. (Initially, the patient on a low-protein diet may be in negative nitrogen balance, but this corrects itself if total caloric intake continues to be adequate.)

To prepare diets containing palatable and readily digestible nonprotein foods that supply calories in the amounts needed requires considerable skill and ingenuity. Daily allowances of appropriate foods for low-protein diets, sample menus based on these restrictions, and special recipes are in the Appendix.

Regulation of various renal functions is usually required for comfort and safety of patients on restricted diets, but these adjustments are of greater significance, of course, for those on the very-low-protein allowances. In addition, various organs, such as those in the cardiovascular and erythropoietic systems, may require therapeutic measures to maintain their activity.

Salt and Water Balance—The manner in which the severely diseased kidney handles sodium may produce excessive hydration on the one hand or dehydration and salt depletion on the other.[3] The control of hydration may require a low-sodium diet, which is often unpalatable, whereas oral salt supplementation may be necessary to arrest or prevent dehydration. In these extreme situations (or even in less severe cases), a normal electrolyte pattern generally cannot be maintained. Therefore, it is necessary to accept whatever appears optimal for the particular patient. Sound medical judgment demands that the whole patient be treated rather than the laboratory report.

Although rigid restriction of sodium intake may be dangerous (the uremia may be aggravated and the acidosis increased because of further depression of the glomerular filtration rate), an excess of sodium may cause a congested state with edema. When edema is present, sodium restriction must be attempted. If marked acidosis develops and also requires control, the kidney's task of excreting acid can be lightened by substitution of appropriate amounts of sodium bicarbonate or lactate for sodium chloride.

Because the severely diseased kidney is unable to produce a concentrated urine, water intake should be adequate to allow excretion of the solute load. However, water in excess may cause a relative hyponatremia, and it must be restricted in acute or terminal uremia or in anuric states.

Potassium—In most cases of chronic renal insufficiency, the potassium level in the blood is normal. In contrast, when chronic renal failure is advanced, blood potassium is commonly elevated. Reduction in oral potassium intake may effectively lower the high levels, but administration of cation-exchange resins orally or as retention enemas will be necessary in some instances.

Calcium and Phosphate—Serum phosphates usually are elevated in advanced renal disease. Restricted intake and phosphate-binding gels may be effective in lowering the high serum concentrations.

In contrast, serum calcium is usually low. When it is normal and the renal disease is advanced, secondary hyperparathyroidism is suggested. If serum calcium is elevated because of parathyroid overactivity or vitamin D therapy, calcium deposition may occur in various tissues. Vitamin D therapy is, therefore, extremely dangerous and should not be used in patients when serum phosphates are high. When such therapy is required (as, for example, in bone disease), it must be preceded by measures that lower phosphates. Some lesions due to calcification disappear when levels of phosphates are brought down.

Anemia—The anemia associated with chronic renal insufficiency is of the normochromic, normocytic type. It is refractory to most forms of therapy because it is due to short red-cell life and depressed red-cell production in the bone marrow, presumably caused by lack of renal erythropoietin. Transfusion of packed red cells poor in buffy coat will benefit patients with symptoms secondary to anemia.

Heart Failure and Hypertension—Treatment of heart failure is essentially the same, irrespective of its cause. When digitalis is used in the presence of renal insufficiency, the usual dose must be reduced because excretion processes in the damaged kidneys are much less efficient. This applies especially to digitoxin.

Hypertension may be difficult to control. Diuretics with hypotensive action may reduce glomerular filtration and thereby aggravate the uremia. However, hypertension in renal disease is reported to respond to some therapeutic measures.[4,5]

Daily Rest—Glomerular filtration rate and renal blood flow are believed to increase in the recumbent position. Accordingly, patients with chronic renal disease should be strongly urged to rest during the day to take advantage of these small but beneficial increases in renal functions.

DIALYSIS

When the glomerular filtration rate falls below 3 ml. per minute, diet therapy no longer can be expected to sustain life, and chronic dialysis (or transplantation, which will be discussed separately) is required.[6] However, it is desirable to begin a program of regular dialysis before this stage is reached—that is, when the glomerular filtration rate is about 3 ml. per minute. Such a precaution is necessary to prevent encephalopathy, cachexia, neuropathy, and bone disorders.

Dialysis may also be a temporary measure. Patients with moderately severe chronic renal insufficiency may need dialysis only on an infrequent but regular basis as well as during transient episodes of reduced renal function.

Two procedures are available—*peritoneal dialysis* and *hemodialysis*. Each technic has its own indications; hence, each may be used with distinct advantages in a given patient, depending on the situation.

Peritoneal Dialysis—The procedure was first performed successfully in 1923 but has been widely used only since 1959. It is considered an effective way to correct uremia, to remove edema fluid as well as exogenous intoxicants (barbiturates or salicylates) and those of endogenous origin (calcium, uric acid, potassium, etc.), and to restore electrolyte balance. Peritoneal dialysis may be preferred during acute renal emergencies—due to surgery, trauma, or infection not involving he abdomen—to maintain the patient until return of residual functions.

The dialysis is carried out in the patient's abdominal cavity with the peritoneum serving as a dialyzing membrane. Only very simple equipment is required. Furthermore, it can be done easily by one person—a physician who is trained in paracentesis and prepared to deal with the problem of maintaining homeostasis.

A stylet catheter is inserted into the abdomen, which is filled with the dialyzing fluid. The withdrawal of fluid from the peritoneal cavity through the catheter is done by siphon action, and refilling is by gravity. Each filling is allowed to equilibrate for twenty to thirty minutes; generally, a patient requires thirty two-liter exchanges each week.

Several types of permanent peritoneal cannulas have been devised during the past decade to accommodate the patient who needs chronic peritoneal dialysis. Experience with them indicates that any prosthesis which remains fixed increases the risk of peritonitis and adhesions. However, a semipermanent (usable less than one year) peritoneal catheter has been developed and is advantageous in patients awaiting more definitive arrangements (hemodialysis or transplantation).

Peritoneal dialysis solutions can be obtained commercially. In addition to the standard formulations, solutions with higher amounts of glucose—i.e., 4.25 or 7 percent rather than 1.5 percent—are available to control overhydration and hypertension. However, the more concentrated glucose solutions increase loss of protein. Also, they may remove more water than sodium, and this tends to increase sodium concentration in the tissues. In some instances, special low-sodium solutions may be required to control hypertension.

The loss of some protein during peritoneal dialysis is undesirable but is unavoidable. Presumably, it occurs because the peritoneal membrane is altered and allows passage of most plasma proteins. Despite protein loss of about 50 Gm. per week, the blood protein can be maintained at normal concentration by adherence to an appropriate nutritional regimen and an occasional intravenous transfusion of plasma.

A second objectionable feature of peritoneal dialysis is its relative inefficiency (about one-fifth to one-tenth that of hemodialysis), although there is improvement when the rate of fluid exchange is increased. To achieve more efficiency, automatic cycling devices are available.

Peritoneal dialysis will continue to play an important role in management of renal insufficiency. It is a simple procedure that is sparing of both equipment and trained people, since the need and resulting hazards of circulating blood outside the patient's body are avoided.

Hemodialysis—In 1947, the purification of blood outside the body was shown by Kolff to be feasible. The early artificial kidney was a cumbersome and expensive machine that did not immediately encourage the widespread use of hemodialysis. Since 1956, development of better machines and their commercial availability have made possible a growing number of dialysis centers throughout the country. In addition, appropriate equipment and training programs are becoming available for hemodialysis in the home.

Two types of commercial artificial kidneys are in general use. In the "coil" design, single or parallel flat cellophane tubes, which may be ten meters long, are wrapped around a central core supported by plastic screening. The dialysis solution is pumped through the concentric layers and over the flattened tubing (Figure 65). The coil assembly can be obtained presterilized and is generally discarded after use.

Since resistance to rapid flow is high, a pump is required to augment the patient's blood flow through the coil. The pressure

Figure 65. Diagram of a simplified coil-type apparatus for hemodialysis. The patient with an A-V shunt is attached to the apparatus, as shown in a. The appearance of the A-V shunt between dialyzing sessions is given in b. The position of the two needles and the direction of blood flow in a patient with an A-V fistula are in c. Blood from the radial artery (light red) is conveyed by pump (d) to the cellophane coil immersed in dialyzing fluid. The fluid, shown in a gray tone, circulates between the layers of the coil, as indicated by arrows. Dialysis takes place during the time the blood is flowing from one end of the coil to the other. When the blood (dark red) leaves the coil, it passes through a clot-and-bubble filter (e) and is then returned to the patient via a wrist vein.

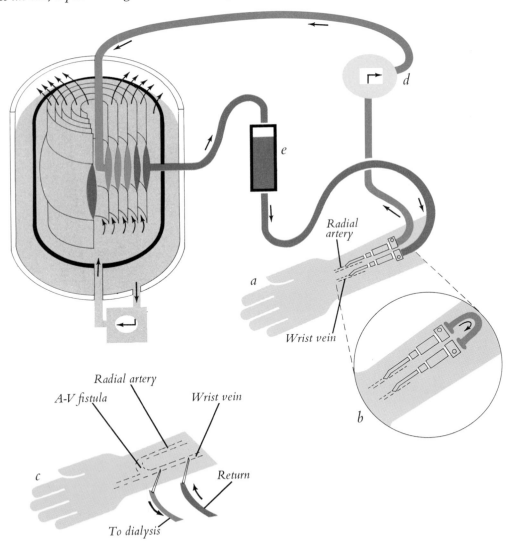

developed by the pump can make the unit function as an ultrafilter as well as a dialyzer.

The efficiency of the augmented-flow coil dialyzer exceeds that of any other dialyzer available; consequently, it is the system of choice when dialysis must be carried out quickly to remove nitrogenous waste substances or toxic materials. However, the presence of the pump introduces potential hazards, and both extensive monitoring and incorporation of safety devices are mandatory.

The "plate," or "layer," dialyzer contains cellophane sheets in place of tubes. These are held slightly apart within plastic frames to allow passage of blood between them. The dialyzing solution flows on the outside of these sheets in a direction opposite to that of the blood. Since resistance to flow is negligible in the plate dialyzer, blood pumping is not necessary. Plate dialyzers are considerably less efficient than the coil types but are relatively trouble-free and require little supervision. All parts that come in contact with the blood are easy to sterilize and are disposable.

With either system, the patient's blood must be conducted to the dialysis unit, purified, and then returned to him. The usual route is via cannulas inserted in the radial artery and a forearm vein. A procedure has been devised which makes it unnecessary to repeat the cannulations for each session in chronic dialysis (Figure 65, a and b). Teflon®-tipped silastic shunts are generally implanted in the radial artery and forearm vein. Both indwelling tubes emerge onto the surface of the arm where they are interconnected by a separate and detachable section of tubing. The "bypass" thus formed allows blood to circulate through the entire prosthesis and prevents clotting. The bypass section is removed when the artery and vein are connected to the artificial kidney and reinserted when dialysis is completed. The arteriovenous shunt may re-main usable without change for a long period, even months or years.

A recent development which allows the patient greater freedom than the external shunt is a surgically prepared subcutaneous A-V fistula involving the radial artery and wrist vein. Each dialysis entails the equivalent of two venipunctures, with needles placed as in Figure 65, c. After the dialyzing session, both needles are removed.

Clotting must be prevented in the dialysis circuit. This may be accomplished by the usual heparinization procedure to prolong clotting time. When systemic anticoagulation is contraindicated, regional heparinization may be employed.

Hemodialysis is now a thoroughly established and definitive treatment for chronic renal failure. Improvements in dialysis equipment—especially development of home dialysis units—as well as refinement of such technics as the arteriovenous shunt are making hemodialysis available to an increasing number of patients.

TRANSPLANTATION

The first successful renal transplantation was performed in 1955 between identical twins.*[7] Transplantation between nonidentical twins was done in 1960 and was soon followed by transplants between individuals with no genetic similarity.[8] Over 3,000 kidney transplants are now on record.

Sources of Kidneys—Kidneys suitable for transplantation may be obtained from living volunteers or cadavers.[9]

When donor selection is evaluated, survival

---

*Transplants of tissue between individuals with identical antigens (i.e., identical twins) are *isografts*. Transplants between genetically dissimilar individuals are *allografts*, formerly called "homografts." If tissue is obtained from a nonhuman source, the transplant is a *xenograft*, or, according to older terminology, a "heterograft."

of transplants indicates that living related-donor kidneys function for longer periods of time than do the cadaver-donor organs.[10] For example, graft survival for two years is greater than 70 percent among recipients of kidneys from living relatives, whereas it is somewhat more than 50 percent for a similar period when the kidneys are taken from unrelated donors, including cadavers. The overall success with cadaver-donor kidneys is very encouraging, and the use of this source is considered well worth continuing.[11,12]

Selection of Donor—The degree of genetic similarity between donor and recipient is one of the more important factors determining the outcome of a transplant. Only in identical twins are transplant antigens identical; dissimilarities exist between all other individuals. They are likely to be of lesser importance when donor and recipient are blood relatives, but, even then, the genetic match will be far from the ideal. Obviously, it should be as similar as possible. Application of appropriate criteria for donor selection is, therefore, of inestimable importance to the success of the transplant.

The degree of genetic similarity between donor and recipient can be estimated by histocompatibility matching procedures.[13,14] This form of genetic typing is based on the observation that transplantation antigens reside on the cell membrane of leukocytes; consequently, these cells can be used for matching between prospective donor and recipient. Typing serums for the growing number of transplantation antigens are now readily available. The technics of the test are standard, and nomenclature on all such antigens is universal. The degree of similarity is judged by comparison of donor-recipient typing. The more nearly alike the antigenic pattern is, the better is the match. In general,

donor cells should not have antigens not also present on the recipient cells, because these can stimulate antibody formation when they are transplanted.

At present, leukocyte typing identifies only a partial list of antigens. Even in the sibling donor-recipient pair who are a "perfect match," sufficient unknown antigenic differences may exist to prevent successful transplantation were it not for methods of immunosuppression. It is hoped that the recipient's reaction to antigens introduced with the donor organ can be suppressed by appropriate drug therapy.

In addition to tests for histocompatibility antigen, the living donor should also receive a variety of tests on the kidneys and the urinary tract. These should include culture of urine, creatinine clearance, intravenous pyelogram, and a renal arteriogram. Donor and recipient should have compatible blood types in order to prevent hemagglutination in the transplanted kidney.

Recipient Selection—The number of patients with terminal renal failure greatly exceeds the number who are selected for transplantation. The successful candidate is one with chronic irreversible renal failure which has advanced to a point where hemodialysis is essential to maintain life. The patient has neither a serious infection nor any systemic disease, such as severe diabetes or generalized arteriosclerosis; that is, he is free of disease which may destroy the new kidney or limit his life. There is no uncorrected abnormality of the lower urinary tract, and the patient is emotionally stable. The latter requirement is frequently difficult to assess in the chronically and often preterminally ill patient. Furthermore, it is essential that he does not have a disease which may be seriously worsened by immunosuppressive and steroid therapy.

The recipient should be brought to the best clinical condition possible before transplantation is attempted. A program of intensive dialysis should be followed for as long as necessary, and hyperkalemia and anemia should be corrected as much as possible. In the patient with pyelonephritis, both kidneys may have to be removed prior to transplantation to eradicate the foci of infection. When glomerulonephritis is present, removal of the kidneys does not necessarily prevent development of glomerulonephritis in the transplanted organ.

Proliferative recurrent glomerulonephritis is the major cause of failure in identical twin recipients and is believed to be due to auto-antibodies against the glomerular basement-membrane antigen. Removal of the recipient's own kidneys does not eliminate these antibodies if they are present. They remain to attack the transplanted kidney and, in the absence of immunosuppressive drugs, continue to be produced. Recurrent glomerulonephritis rarely occurs in nontwin recipients; but, if it does, presumably it is because the glomerular basement-membrane antigens are similar in different individuals.

The selection of transplant recipients remains a difficult problem. In some transplantation centers, the choice of recipients has been assigned to a group of physicians who know the problems but are not personally involved in the care of these patients. Committees of lay members have been used to evaluate prospective recipients on nonmedical grounds.

Surgical Management—The procedure used in transplanting a kidney is not technically difficult, but it must be done in the shortest possible time so that the period of ischemia is kept to a minimum.[15] If delay is unavoidable, it may be helpful to perfuse the kidney with a cooled (10° to 15°C.) electrolyte solution containing procaine and heparin, at a pressure of 70 mm. Hg.

The kidney is usually placed retroperitoneally in the center lateral iliac fossa; the renal artery is anastomosed to the internal iliac artery, and the renal vein to the external, or common, iliac vein. The ureter is shortened to about one-third of its length and tunneled into the bladder.

Medical Management—The major problem encountered in management of transplant patients is adequate but not excessive immunosuppression.

The drugs used most often for immunosuppression are azathioprine and prednisone. Consistent long-term survival of renal transplants began with usage of azathioprine. Leukopenia and thrombocytopenia are hazards, particularly during the initial period when dosages are high. Prednisone is considered most effective for reversal of acute rejection. Side-effects which must be guarded against are acute gastro-intestinal ulceration, psychological changes, diabetes, and demineralization of bone.

The newest and most interesting addition for immunosuppression is antilymphocytic globulin (ALG). ALG is prepared in horses or other animals by injection of lymphocytes from a variety of sources. When administered to patients, it usually produces lymphopenia, but its exact mechanism of action (if it is active at all) is not known.

The Future—Neither of the life-sustaining procedures in chronic renal failure—dialysis or transplantation—has reached such an advanced stage of development that one is clearly superior to the other.

Obviously, regular dialysis, whether at home or in a center, is very time-consuming, since it literally ties the patient to a machine for many hours each week. Its optimum benefits—periods when the plasma is "normal"—persist for only a relatively short time after each session. Even under ideal conditions, the dialysis patient must follow some dietary restrictions and is required to limit his physical activities. In addition, anemia, hypertension, and infection may need persistent therapy. However, in spite of the inefficiency of the method and its inconveniences, the life expectancy for a dialysis patient at the present time is somewhat longer than that for the average transplant patient. Improvements in machines and technics are constantly being made and will continue to give the dialysis patient greater convenience and comfort as well as safety.

The successful transplant patient may enjoy an entirely normal life, at least for a period of time. Duration of the transplant, however, is unpredictable. Hume and others believe that today's recipient of a related-donor kidney has at least an 85 percent chance of living with that kidney indefinitely.[16,17]

Supplies of kidneys suitable for transplantation are limited; consequently, recipients must be selected from a number of potential candidates. The more extensive use of cadaver kidneys will bring transplantation to many more patients. Developments needed possibly include rapid computer selection of appropriate recipients from a group of co-operating hospitals, effective preservation methods, and uniform laws governing cadaver organs.

Advances in immunosuppressive therapy may involve procedures to modify both the transplant's antigens and the recipient's immunologic response. By these means, the graft will be made less "foreign" and the recipient's reaction less destructive. Furthermore, it may be possible to suppress only those cells engaged in rejection without affecting the cells active in protecting the host from infection. This may perhaps be done with a serum containing the appropriate antibodies or a drug possessing a high degree of specificity.

Many problems, both in dialysis and transplantation, still remain to be solved. However, new technics of research are providing the needed answers at a rapid rate.

BIBLIOGRAPHY

1. Berlyne, G. M.: Nutrition in Renal Disease. Baltimore: The Williams & Wilkins Company, 1968.

2. Giordano, C., Esposito, R., de Pascale, C., and de Santo, N. G.: Dietary Treatment in Renal Failure, Proceedings of the Third International Congress of Nephrology (edited by E. L. Becker), 3:214. New York: S. Karger, 1967.

3. Giovannetti, S.: Diet in Chronic Uremia, Proceedings of the Third International Congress of Nephrology (edited by E. L. Becker), 3:230. New York: S. Karger, 1967.

4. Page, I. H., and Dustan, H. P.: Drug Treatment of Arterial Hypertension. New York: American Heart Association, 1969.

5. Page, I. H., and McCubbin, J. W.: Renal Hypertension. Chicago: Year Book Medical Publishers, Inc., 1968.

6. Merrill, J. P.: The Treatment of Renal Failure; Therapeutic Principles in the Management of Acute and Chronic Uremia, Ed. 2. New York: Grune & Stratton, Inc., 1965.

7. Murray, J. E., Merrill, J. P., and Harrison, J. H.: Homotransplantation in Identical Twins, S. Forum, 6:432, 1955.

8. Merrill, J. P., Murray, J. E., Harrison, J. H., Friedman, E. A., Dealy, J. B., Jr., and Dammin, G. J.: Successful Homotransplantation of the Kidney between Nonidentical Twins, New England J. Med., *262*:1251, 1960.

9. Murray, J. E., Barnes, B. A., and Atkinson, J.: Fifth Report of the Human Kidney Transplant Registry, Transplantation, *5*:752, 1967.

10. Starzl, T. E., Marchioro, T. L., Terasaki, P. I., Porter, K. A., Faris, T. D., Herrmann, T. J., Vredevoe, D. L., Hutt, M. P., Ogden, D. A., and Waddell, W. R.: Chronic Survival after Human Renal Homotransplantation; Lymphocyte-Antigen Matching, Pathology and Influence of Thymectomy, Ann. Surg., *162*:749, 1965.

11. Straffon, R. A., Stewart, B. H., Kiser, W. S., *et al.*: The Use of Ninety-Four Cadaveric Kidneys for Transplantation—Clinical Experience, Brit. J. Urol., *38*:640, 1966.

12. Hume, D. M., Lee, H. M., Williams, G. M., White, H. J. O., Ferré, J., Wolf, J. S., Prout, G. R., Jr., Slapak, M., O'Brien, J., Kilpatrick, S. J., Kauffman, H. M., Jr., and Cleveland, R. J.: Comparative Results of Cadaver and Related Donor Renal Homografts in Man, and Immunologic Implications of the Outcome of Second and Paired Transplants, Ann. Surg., *164*:352, 1966.

13. Brent, L., and Medawar, P. B.: Tissue Transplantation: A New Approach to the "Typing" Problem, Brit. M. J., *2*:269, 1963.

14. Murray, J. E., and Harrison, J. H.: Surgical Management of Fifty Patients with Kidney Transplants Including Eighteen Pairs of Twins, Am. J. Surg., *105*:205, 1963.

15. Abaza, H. M., Nolan, B., Watt, J. G., and Woodruff, M. F. A.: Effect of Antilymphocytic Serum on the Survival of Renal Homotransplants in Dogs, Transplantation, *4*:618, 1966.

16. Hume, D. M.: Progress in Clinical Renal Homotransplantation, Advances Surg., *2*:419, 1966.

17. Hamburger, J., Crosnier, J., and Dormont, J.: Experience with 45 Renal Homotransplantations in Man, Lancet, *1*:985, 1965.

GENERAL REFERENCES

Becker, E. L. (Editor): Structural Basis of Renal Disease. New York: Hoeber Medical Division, Harper & Row, Publishers, 1968.

Black, D. A. K. (Editor): Renal Disease, Ed. 2. Philadelphia: F. A. Davis Company, 1967.

Brest, A. N., and Moyer, J. H. (Editors): Renal Failure. Philadelphia: J. B. Lippincott Company, 1967.

Hamburger, J., Richet, G., Crosnier, J., Funck-Brentano, J. L., Antoine, B., Ducrot, H., Méry, J. P., and de Montera, H.: Nephrology. Philadelphia: W. B. Saunders Company, 1968.

Heptinstall, R. H.: Pathology of the Kidney. Boston: Little, Brown & Company, 1966.

Kass, E. H. (Editor): Progress in Pyelonephritis. Philadelphia: F. A. Davis Company, 1965.

Pitts, R. F.: Physiology of the Kidney and Body Fluids, Ed. 2. Chicago: Year Book Medical Publishers, Inc., 1968.

Schreiner, G. E., and Maher, J. F.: Uremia: Biochemistry, Pathogenesis and Treatment, p. 487. Springfield, Illinois: Charles C Thomas, Publisher, 1961.

Strauss, M. B., and Welt, L. G. (Editors): Diseases of the Kidney. Boston: Little, Brown & Company, 1963.

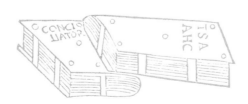

APPENDIX

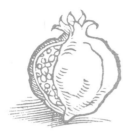

Foods for Low-Protein Diets (No Meat or Fish)

Daily Allowances	*Daily Allowances*

Milk, whole. . . . . 1/2 cup
(Omit skim milk, buttermilk, yogurt, ice cream, cheese.)

Eggs . . . . 1 egg
Prepared in any way or used in cooking

Fats . . . . As desired
Butter, margarine, oils, vegetable shortening
(Omit salad dressings, mayonnaise, gravy.)

Bread, wheat starch . . . . As desired
It is best toasted and eaten with butter and jam.

Bread, white . . . . 2 slices
(Omit all other commercial breads, biscuits, muffins, pancakes, crackers.)

Pastries, wheat starch . . . . As desired
Muffins, cookies, etc.
(Omit all commercial pastries.)

Cereals, cooked . . . . 1/2 cup
Any cooked or quick-cooked cereal, tapioca, polished rice, macaroni, noodles, spaghetti (made with water or the milk allowance)
(Omit brown and wild rice.)

Cereals, dry . . . . 1/2 cup
Cornflakes, Rice Krispies, Puffed Rice, Shredded Wheat, Cheerios, Wheaties, Rice Chex, Wheat Chex, Bran Flakes, Frosted Flakes, All-Bran, Raisin Bran, Sugar Smacks
(Omit all other cereals.)

Vegetables, cooked. . . . . 1 cup
Fresh, frozen, or canned (unsalted) asparagus, beets, cabbage, carrots, cucumbers, eggplant, green beans, green pepper, lettuce, mushrooms, onions, potatoes, radishes, squash, tomatoes, turnips, wax beans
Broccoli, Brussels sprouts, corn, and spinach are *high-protein* vegetables and should be eaten only twice a week.
(Omit all other vegetables.)

Soup . . . . 1 cup
Unsalted homemade vegetable or potato soup *without meat*
(Omit all commercial canned, frozen, or dehydrated soups.)

Vegetable juices . . . . As desired

Fruits and juices . . . . 2 1/2 cups
All fresh, frozen, dried, and canned fruits or juices
Ices made with frozen fruit juices or puddings prepared with fruit or fruit juice and tapioca

Sweeteners . . . . As desired
Sugar (brown and white), honey, jam, jelly, maple syrup, marshmallows

Condiments and spices . . . . As desired
Onion or garlic powder, pepper, herbs, chives, lemon juice, vinegar, parsley, food flavorings
(Omit salt, seasoned salt, monosodium glutamate, allspice, catsup, mustard; pickles, relishes, olives, etc., with salt.)

Soft drinks . . . . As desired

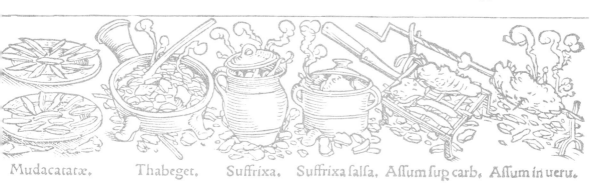

Mudacaratæ.   Thabeget.   Suffrixa.   Suffrixa falfa.   Affum fup carb.   Affum in ueru.

Sample Menus (Approximately 40 Gm. of Protein)

Breakfast	Lunch	Dinner

Apricot nectar
Oatmeal, brown sugar
Toast, butter, jam
Milk
Coffee, sugar
	Vegetable plate:
	    Scrambled egg, buttered carrots
	    and asparagus tips, home-fried
	    potatoes
	Toast, butter, jelly
	Cola drink
	
	Snack (3:00 p.m.)
	Lemonade, sugar
	Wheat starch muffin, butter, jelly
		Fruit plate:
		    Pears, plums, applesauce
		Wheat starch bread, butter
		Water ice
		Tea, sugar
		
		Snack (8:00 p.m.)
		Fruit juice, sugar

Cranberry juice
Rice Krispies, banana, milk, sugar
Wheat starch toast, butter,
    marmalade
Tea, sugar
	Homemade potato soup
	Hard-cooked egg, lettuce, tomato
	    on white toast
	Baked apple
	Ginger ale
	
	Snack (3:00 p.m.)
	Tea, honey, lemon
	Wheat starch bread, butter, jelly
		Baked potato, butter
		Buttered corn
		Cucumber, oil, vinegar
		Wheat starch bread, butter
		Tapioca fruit pudding
		Tea, sugar
		
		Snack (8:00 p.m.)
		Apple cider
		Wheat starch cookies

Stewed prunes Cream of Rice Wheat starch muffin, butter, jelly Milk (1/4 cup) Tea, sugar	French toast (2 slices bread, 1 egg, 1/4 cup milk) Maple syrup Minted pineapple slices Fruit punch *Snack (3:00 p.m.)* Cornstarch pudding	Baked sweet potato, marshmallow Buttered green beans Tossed salad, oil, vinegar Wheat starch bread, butter Tea, sugar *Snack (8:00 p.m.)* Fruitade, lemonade, or grape juice

Peach nectar
Cornflakes, milk, brown sugar
Toast, butter, honey
Coffee, sugar
	Poached egg on toast
	Parslied buttered potato
	Buttered green beans
	Cola drink
	
	Snack (3:00 p.m.)
	Ginger ale float
	    (made with water ice)
		Fruit plate:
		    Peaches, bananas, cherries
		Wheat starch muffin, butter, jam
		Milk
		Tea, sugar
		
		Snack (8:00 p.m.)
		Grape juice, sugar
		Wheat starch bread, butter, jelly

Some Recipes for Low-Protein Diets

Low-Protein Bread

1 1/4 cups warm water (100°F.)
1 package active dry yeast
4 tablespoons sugar
1/2 teaspoon double-acting baking powder
 (or 3/4 teaspoon sodium-free baking powder*)
1 teaspoon salt (or none*)
2 3/4 cups Paygel P Wheat Starch
1/4 cup hydrogenated shortening

Procedure

1. Place water, yeast, and 1 tablespoon of sugar in large mixing bowl. Stir until yeast dissolves.
2. Let stand for 5 minutes before adding dry ingredients and shortening.
3. Moisten ingredients at low speed; then mix for 1 minute at high speed, scraping only sides of bowl with rubber spatula.
4. Cover with towel and leave at room temperature for 30 minutes.
5. Beat mixture about 50 strokes and pour into a greased loaf pan (9″ x 5″ x 2 3/4″ or 8 1/2″ x 4 1/2″ x 2 5/8″).
6. Cover and let stand for an additional 30 minutes.
7. Bake for 55 minutes at 375°F.

Note: If mixture resembles piecrust, add 1 or 2 tablespoons of water; if it is like pancake batter, add same amount of wheat starch.

Rhubarb Pudding

2 cups canned sweetened rhubarb
1/2 cup water
1/3 cup sugar

---
*When diet must also be low in sodium.

2 drops red food coloring
1 level tablespoon cornstarch
2 tablespoons water

Procedure

1. Add 1/2 cup water, sugar, and food coloring to rhubarb and bring to a boil.
2. Stir in cornstarch mixed with 2 tablespoons of water and cook for 2 minutes.
3. Add vanilla, if desired.
4. Pour into 4 serving cups and top with 2 tablespoons of heavy cream.

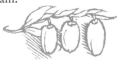

Lemon Cookies
(approximately 5 dozen)

1/2 cup hydrogenated shortening
1 cup brown sugar, packed
1 egg yolk
 (or 1 tablespoon lemon juice)
1 tablespoon lemon rind
1 1/2 cups Paygel P Wheat Starch
1/2 teaspoon baking soda
1/2 teaspoon cream of tartar
1/4 teaspoon ginger
Granulated sugar

Procedure

1. Mix shortening, brown sugar, and egg yolk (or lemon juice); then add lemon rind.
2. Blend in dry ingredients.
3. Roll rounded teaspoons of dough into balls and dip tops in granulated sugar.
4. Place on ungreased cookie sheet and bake for 10 to 12 minutes at 350°F.

Wheat Starch Muffins

1 1/2 cups wheat starch flour
2 teaspoons double-acting baking powder
  (*or* 3 teaspoons sodium-free baking powder*)
2 tablespoons honey
2 tablespoons salad oil
1/4 cup canned applesauce
1/4 cup half and half
1/2 cup water
1 tablespoon sugar

Procedure

1. Sift flour, baking powder, and sugar together into mixing bowl.
2. Combine applesauce, honey, and oil and mix into dry ingredients.
3. Add half and half and water; stir until the mixture is well blended.
4. Pour into lightly greased muffin tin and bake at 375°F. for 25 to 30 minutes.

Blueberry Muffins
(12 muffins)

1/4 cup butter
1/2 cup sugar
3 tablespoons water
1/2 teaspoon vanilla
2 teaspoons double-acting baking powder
  (*or* 3 teaspoons sodium-free baking powder*)
3/4 cup plus 2 tablespoons Paygel P Wheat Starch

----
*When diet must also be low in sodium.

1 egg white, stiffly beaten
1/2 cup fresh or frozen, thawed, and drained blueberries.

Procedure

1. Preheat oven to 375°F.
2. Cream butter and sugar.
3. Add water, vanilla, and dry ingredients and mix thoroughly.
4. Fold in egg white and blueberries.
5. Pour batter into greased muffin tin and bake for 25 to 30 minutes.

Note: Muffins do not turn golden brown.

Herb Toast

Suggested Herbs and Seasonings
Onion powder
Garlic powder
Toasted sesame seed
Poppy seed
Dillseed
Anise seed
Caraway seed
Chives

Procedure

1. Preheat oven to 500°F.
2. Slice low-protein bread 3/8 inch thick.
3. Bake the slices of bread for 3 minutes or until dry but not brown.
4. Turn slices over, spread with butter (unsalted*), and then sprinkle with herbs or seasoning.
5. Bake for 4 minutes or until brown.

INDEX

60-PQ-0027-2   PRINTED IN U.S.A.   400681-77450   JULY, 1974